DR. SUSAN R. CUSHING
Award Winning Author of FAT NO MORE! THE BOOK OF HOPE FOR LOSING WEIGHT

HAVE NO FEAR
OF THE DENTAL CHAIR!
A GUIDE FOR REDUCING DENTAL FEAR

Includes a Captivating Prologue on *My Story and My Mission*

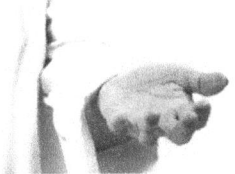

Never be afraid of the dentist anymore.

Includes 19 Cases of Neuro-Linguistic Programming Success!

For Dental Patients and Professionals

╬RICHER Press
An Imprint of Richer Life, LLC

RICHER Press is a full service, specialty Trade publisher whose sole goal is to *shape thoughts and change lives for the better.* All of the books, eBooks and digital media we publish, distribute and market embrace our commitment to help maximize opportunities for personal growth and professional achievement.

To learn more visit
www.richerlifellc.com

Publisher's Disclaimer

This book does not provide medical advice.

The information, including but not limited to, text, graphics, images and other material, contained in this book is for educational and inspirational purposes only. The content is not intended in any way as a substitute for professional medical advice, diagnosis or treatment. Always seek the advice of your physician or other qualified healthcare provider with any questions you may have regarding a medical condition or treatment and before undertaking a new health care regimen, and never disregard professional medical advice or delay in seeking it because of something you have read in this book.

Copyright © 2016 by Susan R. Cushing

Published by ✠RICHER Press
An Imprint of Richer Life, LLC

4600 E. Washington Street, Suite 300, Phoenix, Arizona 85034
www.richerlifellc.com

Cover Design: RICHER Media USA

No part of this publication may be reproduced, stored in a retrieval system, or transmitted in any form or by any means, electronic, mechanical, photocopying, recording, scanning, or otherwise, except as permitted under Section 107 or 108 of the 1976 United States Copyright Act, without prior written permission of the publisher.

Library of Congress Cataloging-in-Publications Data

Have No Fear of the Dental Chair!
A Guide for Reducing Dental Fear

Susan R. Cushing
p.   cm.

1. Dentistry 2. Self Help 3. Inspiration
ISBN 978-0-9970831-0-1
(pbk : alk. Paper)

2014935145

ISBN 13: 978-0-9970831-0-1
ISBN 10: 0-9970831-0-7

Text set is Adobe Garamond

PRINTED IN THE UNITED STATES OF AMERICA

March 2016

CONTENTS

DEDICATION   11

ACKNOWLEDGEMENTS   13

PROLOGUE   15

From Fearful Patient to Dental Professional and Anti-Anxiety Advocate
My Story and My Mission

- **How Did I End Up Here?**
- **My First Dental Visit**
  The Pain and the Unpleasant Memories
- **My Second Dental Visit**
  More Pain, More Promises and Perceived Vulnerabilities
- **Maturity, Braces and Smiling Dentists**
  A New Path for My Life
- **Beyond Fearful Child To Dental School**
- **Obtaining Clinical Skills, Helping Patients and Becoming an Anti-Anxiety Advocate**

  · Discovering Techniques and Seeing Fearful Patients Respond

  · Becoming an Anti-Anxiety Advocate

  · How This Book Can Help You

A GUIDE FOR REDUCING DENTAL FEAR

Chapter 1	Understanding Dental Fear and Common Fears of a Dental Patient What is the Dental Profession Saying?	43
Chapter 2	Common Anesthetics and Pain Prevention	55
Chapter 3	The Reasons Patients Schedule Appointments	65
Chapter 4	Anxiety Reducing Tools	69
Chapter 5	Hypnosis and Acupuncture	91
Chapter 6	Barriers to Getting Dental Care for Fearful Patients Why are the Statistics of People Afraid to go to the Dentist Still So High?	97
Chapter 7	Specific Needs of a Fearful Dental Patient	101
Chapter 8	What Can Lead To or Turn into Dental Anxiety? Fear Responses and Triggers	105
Chapter 9	What Can Anxious Patients Do to Prepare for a Dental Appointment?	111
Chapter 10	What Can Anxious Patients Do to Help Themselves at the Dental Appointment?	117

Chapter 11	Gagging	123
Chapter 12	Childhood Dental Trauma Simplest and Most Effective Tools Available	129
Chapter 13	Using NLP For Dental Anxiety with the Phobic Patient	135
Chapter 14	Selecting the Techniques That are Best for You	141

GLOSSARY OF TERMS	145
REFERENCES	155
NINETEEN NLP CASES AND TWO INTERESTING STORIES	157
PATIENT LETTERS AND TESTIMONIALS	227
ABOUT THE AUTHOR	233

Dedication

I dedicate this book to my mother, Evelyn Cushing, who never really understood me, but did the best she could. She worked very hard to find a way to get me the dental care I needed.

And also to Dr. Albert Puccia, whose kindness and compassion took a terrified teenager (me) and helped her overcome her dental fear, whereby saving her teeth and inspiring her toward her profession and her mission.

HAVE NO FEAR OF THE DENTAL CHAIR!

Acknowledgements

I want to thank my publisher and editor, Earl Cobb, for being an amazing mentor and friend, my dearest friends, Alice, Rachel, Mary Ann, Sandra, Jeannie, Nancy and Phil who have inspired me to be the best I can be and all those that have been there for me throughout the years.

Most of all I want to acknowledge and thank my husband, Curt, who has always loved me unconditionally and encouraged me in all my endeavors.

HAVE NO FEAR OF THE DENTAL CHAIR!

PROLOGUE

FROM FEARFUL PATIENT TO ANTI-ANXIETY ADVOCATE

My Story and My Mission

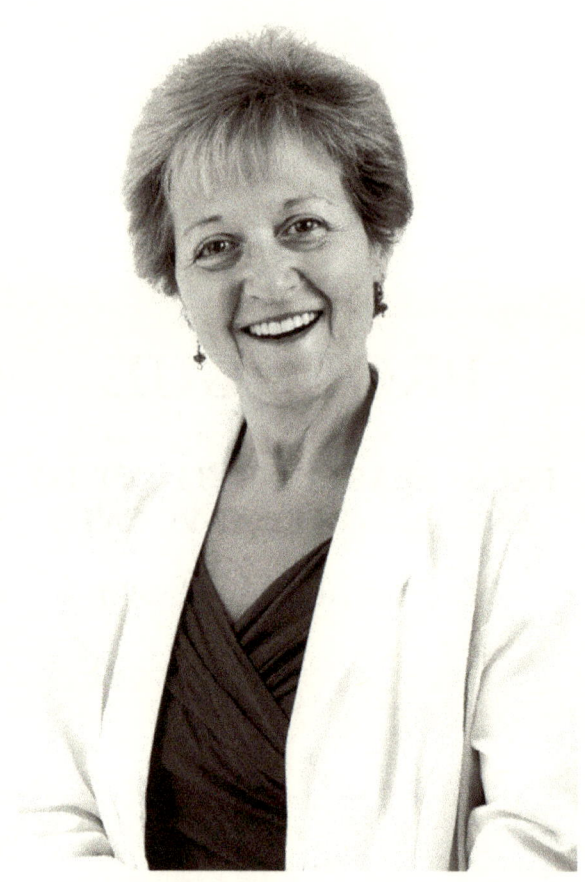

"My first memory of anything dental was having a dental exam at my elementary school and being told I had cavities."

HOW DID I END UP HERE?

How did I end up here? Good question, you say. Excellent question is what I reply.

Well, let me tell you about what I can remember and what the entire subject of dentistry was like for me.

As a child and young teen, all the way up to my thirties, I had an unrelenting "sweet tooth." I just loved candy, gum, cookies, cake and soda. The more I could get and the faster I could get it into my mouth, the better.

It began as an enjoyable and tasty treat, a moment in time, but it became an obsession and ultimately an addiction. I might have even "mainlined" the sugar if I had the option!

I would eat rock candy (pure sugar made into hard crystals) and frozen Charleston Chew bars till they broke my teeth. I chewed Beeman's & Wrigley's sugared gum and drank bottles of root beer soda till my teeth rotted out. I ate handfuls of cookies, batches of brownies and packages of popsicles. I only stopped when the boxes were empty.

I really do not remember how much I brushed my teeth or even if I did. I idolized sweets and adored candy. I always had some in my pockets, school desk, book bag and purse. I had it squirreled away wherever I could hide it; to be retrieved whenever I wanted it or needed some for comfort.

I have noticed over the years that most kids like sweets when given the opportunity to have some, but I would search them out and eat them any chance I got.

AUTHOR'S NOTE: See my first book, "Fat No More! The Book of Hope for Losing Weight", for details on my sugar & flour and food addiction.

My first memory of anything dental was having a dental exam at my elementary school and being told I had cavities. I must have been a little scared, but I really didn't understand what it meant. It was mostly a fear of the unknown and not of anything in particular.

My parents were notified of my cavities by a letter sent home from school and I was taken to a dental clinic. I truly cannot remember the experience, except that I was hurt by the male dentist and that I cried a lot and was told by the dentist that it "did not hurt that bad". That began the fearful reality for me that dentists hurt people and they deny my reality.

I know that this experience happened more than one time, but I seem to have conveniently blocked it out. I was a young child of six or seven and forgetting was probably a protective mechanism for me.

I do remember, however, that it became an "anchor" experience for me and that I made a conscious decision at age seven that I would rather have the elusive cavity than have a dentist inflict pain on me. As a result there were no more dental appointments; at least for a while.

However, when I went for the next school dental exam, I was told I needed fillings. I had broken a back molar eating my rock candy and made the mistake of telling my teacher that it hurt. When I got home with the school note, I was already crying. I told my mother in a loud voice, "I am not going and you can't make me"…believing I had control of the situation.

MY FIRST DENTAL VISIT
The Pain and the Unpleasant Memories

MY mother told me I had to get it fixed and she would take me to her dentist. My mom had never spoken about her dentist, so I agreed to get into the car.

As my mom parked the car, I could already feel my body tremble and my eyes getting moist. When we got out of the car, she took my hand and we went into her dentist's building. As much as I had tried to hold it in, I couldn't any longer and I exploded. By the time we reached his office. I had tears pouring from my eyes, which soaked the front of my shirt, had a completely stuffed up nose and a very sore throat.

My mother opened the outside door and we walked upstairs to his office, I was overtaken by a terrible smell. When my mother opened his office door, it was even stronger. Inside an older woman was standing up at the end of a long corridor handing something to a man in a white coat.

She looked out at us and then resumed what she had been doing. I could hear someone spitting and coughing and lots of gurgling noises coming from down the hall. I tried very hard not to think about what would happen to me when I got into that room, but I couldn't help it. I got more and more afraid.

Eventually she came out and greeted us and said we would be next. Then, the man in the white coat, who introduced himself as the dentist, said it was my turn and asked us to follow the woman into a small room. I wanted to be brave and for them to like me, but my body was shaking uncontrollably.

I was directed to lie down in this long blue chair and open my mouth so he could do his exam. As he came closer to me, I could smell stale cigarettes and another pungent odor coming from him. I noticed that his hands seemed to be shaking as he put things in my mouth. I was shaking all over and couldn't really determine if it was him or me.

As I looked around the room, I saw a huge blue machine of some kind that resembled a mechanical robot. It had pulleys, wires and all sorts of cords attached and hanging from it. I was soon to learn that this was where his drills, water and suction came from. On the right side of the room I saw a tall chest of what seemed like hundreds of small drawers. I could only imagine what was inside each of them.

However, when I peered over to the far left, I saw this tall glass jar filled with a bluish liquid that contained the biggest needle I had ever seen! That did it for me. I began to cry hysterically until the dentist surprised me by sharply telling me to "stop it, and sit still, so I can finish my exam!"

He spoke over me and told my mother that I had a fractured baby molar that needed to come out and some cavities. Before I could protest and say anything, he came at me with this huge, long needle and stuck it into my mouth until I screamed. The older lady, whom I later learned was his wife and his dental assistant, held me down while he pulled out my tooth. It was over before I knew it, but he had already caused the emotional damage. I had been terrorized, hurt and traumatized, at least in my mind.

He gave my mother the post-operative instructions and told me to bite down on the gauze in my mouth. I could already see blood and saliva dripping along my chin and I continued to cry and shake.

He then told my mother that I had a cavity in the tooth next to the one he pulled out and possibly some others and that I needed to come back for the fillings. The lady gave me a lollypop and we left the office as I continued to cry all the way home. I hated the numb feeling in my lip and ended up playing with it so much that I bit myself and had pain for the next few days.

I spent the next week worrying about going back and imagining that it would be even worse the next time. I had no idea what a filling was, but I was sure that it was terrible and was going to hurt me.

My mother told me that I had to get my cavities filled before they got worse and caused me pain. I fought with her all week. She promised that the next appointment would be better and I would not need a needle.

MY SECOND DENTAL VISIT
More Pain, More Promises and Perceived Vulnerabilities

So, we went back the next week and I told him I did not want a needle. He told me he had to get the tooth numb and when I cried and screamed in protest, his wife held me down again while he used that really long needle.

Then, he put these big drills in my mouth that made me vibrate and shake and feel horrible. He filled the cavities and told me to rinse and spit out. But when I did, I drooled all over myself and saw blood, saliva and some metal stuff coming out into the whirling porcelain spittoon bowl. It was disgusting and even worse than I had imagined.

My mother had lied to me again! It was not better and he did use that huge needle. That awful experience taught me two lessons: (1) I can never tell anyone about my teeth, and (2) I cannot trust my mother to be honest with me where doctors are concerned or to protect me from being hurt.

Let me add here that, as a young child of six years old, I had many sore throats due to infected tonsils and adenoids and had to be taken to the Children's Hospital in Boston. My mother would tell me they were going to make me feel better and at the end of every appointment I was given a shot in my buttocks. When I cried and told my mother that I would not go back if they were going to give me a shot, she would assure me that she would tell the doctor and he would not give me one the next time. However, they always gave me a shot. I had begun to not believe her back then, but hoped that it would be different with the dentist.

After the experiences with her dentist, I realized that my mother would lie to me to get me to go to the hospital or to the dentist. I didn't have the adult understanding or maturity to realize that she was doing what she thought she had to do, so I would get well. My mother had no clue as to how terrifying a needle was to me and what her actions had created in me.

Well, from that moment on, I began to keep my thoughts to myself about many things, especially anything about my teeth.

Thinking back, I remember being told by the school nurse that candy causes cavities, but it was all a big mystery to me. I was told to brush my teeth hard and until the gums bled, which they always did. I hated seeing blood coming out of my mouth, so I think I probably did not brush very often. I was also told to stop eating so much candy and I wouldn't get any cavities. Well, I could accept that I needed to brush occasionally, but not eating any candy was ludicrous and was not going to happen.

How could I possibly ever stop eating something that not only tasted good, but also made me feel so good and actually made me happy?

AUTHOR'S NOTE: Dear Readers - If you have children, please do not make promises that you know you cannot keep... not if you want to develop a trusting relationship with them. Find other strategies to help them calm down and deal with their anxieties. These may include counseling, desensitization, EMDR or Eye Movement Desensitization and Reprocessing, NLP or Neuro-Linguistic Programming, hypnosis, meditation, sedation or whatever else you can add to your "bag of tricks." Find some way to help them through times like these, but not at the expense of your precious relationship. You may think that the end justifies the means in accomplishing the goal. But I can assure you that, from my experience, it will be at too great a cost. I have learned that lying has never been a benefit to me.

Today I know that my mom did the best she could. I believe that my screaming probably made her skin crawl and she worried about me getting sicker, so she lied and told me I would not get the dreaded shot. In truth, she knew all along that I would need another shot of antibiotics to get me well and she hoped that in time I would just forget about it. She seemed to have had very few resources to deal with her frightened little girl but loved me enough to seek help and risk my response.

However, for this sensitive child, me, it was the worst thing my mother could have done. I eventually stopped believing anything she told me. I developed an enormous fear of all doctors in white coats and learned not to trust anybody or anything. It has taken me many, many years to work through this and get beyond it.

MATURITY, BRACES AND SMILING DENTISTS
A New Path for My Life

Now, I will fast forward to Junior High, when our neighbor told my mother that I should get braces. My smile was odd since my top front teeth went under my bottom front teeth and looked funny. Our neighbor's daughter had been going to an orthodontist. So, she gave my mother his name.

In retrospect, I can see just how fortunate I really was and how much my parents, especially my mother, must have loved me. This was the time when most of the families we knew did not send their children to orthodontists due to the cost and the fact that was not the norm for "average" folks like us. Only those with financial resources available and those children with severe malocclusions were regularly sent for treatment. There was no dental insurance and certainly not the widespread dental awareness of dental health that we have today.

My father was a taxi driver and my mom was a bookkeeper at a hospital. Neither of my parents made a very good salary. Certainly not a salary that could provide their family with much more than anything other than the basics: food, shelter and essential medical care. Orthodontics was considered a luxury of those wealthier than we were. My parents worked extremely hard to raise their three children with the primary goal of providing the basics and any opportunity for a better life than they had had. Their primary focus was to keep us healthy and get us a good education.

My father never completed high school, since he had to drop out and work in his father's convenience store, in order to help financially. My mother took the business track at high school so she could become a secretary in order to help contribute to her family. Fortunately, she was good with math and numbers and was able to get a job as a bookkeeper. A job that she loved until the day she retired.

I knew that my mom worked really hard each month to budget what we could afford with paying the bills and keeping us afloat. I remember my mom talking with my dad one night saying that somehow they would find a way to get money to allow me to go to an Orthodontist.

I realize now what a sacrifice it was for both of them to somehow pull out a little money each month to have their "Little Suzy" be able to get braces. If it wasn't for her determination and finesse with budgeting, I would most likely have lost all of my teeth when I reached adulthood and would be wearing upper and lower full dentures.

I am unable to thank her now, since she's been gone for many years, but I can send her love and gratitude to wherever she rests. I do pay it forward by spending a lot of energy helping others save their teeth when possible. I do not want my patients ending up as "dental cripples."

So, because of my mother, I was off to my first orthodontist visit.

I had an enormous amount of anxiety about this whole braces thing, but when I got to the office and sat in the waiting room, I heard no screaming, no crying and no drills. Although my mother had told me this before we got there, I was still wary and did not fully trust her. I knew I had to wait and see it for myself.

When it was my turn, the receptionist called my name and sat me in a room with a chair that reminded me of getting a haircut. The first thing I did when I got into the room was to look around and be sure there were no drills or needles. Not seeing any allowed me to calm down a little until the dentist came into the room. His stiff, long white coat reminded me of the Children's Hospital doctors who treated me when my tonsil's kept getting infected. My mother had to bring me there many times until I finally got my tonsils and adenoids removed.

I am sure that was when most of my needle phobia began. I would have these terrible sore throats and unrelenting earaches and my mother would take me out of school and bring me to the hospital. Every time the doctors would examine me they would tell me my tonsils were infected and then give me a shot in my buttocks. I began to get so hyped up and uncontrollable whenever my mom mentioned that we were going to the hospital. I would cry and scream pleading with her and begging her not to make me go. She would end up promising me the doctors would not give me a shot just to get me to go into the car. However, as I mentioned earlier, the doctors still gave me a shot for my swollen tonsils, while I was screaming hysterically.

As I look back, the worst part of the entire experience was my mother promising me something that she and I both knew she could not keep. It made me turn against her and trust her less and less the older I got. It made me feel unsafe and unprotected and vulnerable.

So, there I was feeling panicked as I stared at this dentist in a long, white coat who only wanted to examine my teeth. I started to cry and go into hysterics. He and his assistant came over to my side and reassured me that he would not hurt me and that he was only going to look at my teeth.

I could see that he only had a mirror in his hand and no needles of any kind, so I opened my mouth tentatively. As I did this, I could feel and taste my tears dropping into my mouth. The dentist, called an orthodontist, said something to his assistant and then began to talk to my mother and me.

He said that I had an under-bite and that he wanted me to go home, take some wooden sticks and put them under my top front teeth. He wanted me to try to push them over my lower front teeth. He said he hoped the sticks might move my teeth forward and where they belonged in about six months or so. He then gave me a mirror, took one of the wooden stick, placed it in my mouth and had me watch in the mirror while he showed me what to do. It was easy and did not hurt at all.

My mother thanked him, paid the receptionist and I was given a lollypop. We both left there without much fuss and I had had my first non-traumatic dental appointment.

I was so relieved that he didn't hurt me and I did not want to have to go back, so I did exactly what he told me to do as many times a day as I could. I bit on those sticks, actually tongue depressors, constantly.

Well, about a year went by and nothing changed. His office was pretty far away and my mother was upset that she did not see any results. So, she asked her friends at work and was given a referral to another orthodontist. This one was easier to get to and my mother made an appointment for me to get a second opinion.

This visit I was not too worried, since the last orthodontist hadn't hurt me and I figured this one wouldn't either. By this time, I also had some classmates wearing braces and they told me braces really didn't hurt much. They told me there's a lot of pressure when they put them on and the wires can cut your lips but then you put wax on and it's fine. I was reassured, by all of them, that there were no needles or drills to cause any pain.

So, off my mother and I went to meet this new orthodontist. When I went into his office, he greeted me with a smile and seemed pretty nice. He looked at my teeth and took some molds of my mouth with stuff that almost made me gag. He told my mother that I had an under bite and I would need a bite plane to help my top teeth go over my bottom teeth followed by a few years of braces. I learned that even though there were no needles or drills in his office, that there were still some awful things that happened, like gagging, but they were bearable to me.

He told my mother that he noticed some cavities that needed to be taken care of before he could start my orthodontic treatment. Also, some teeth would need to be removed to allow him to correct my under-bite.

Well, as you might have expected, the tears and crying began and only got worse once we got into our car. My mother told me she had spoken with him about my fear of needles and he gave her the name of a dentist that used something called "laughing gas" and had a great reputation for treating children with success. She also told me that the assistant had told her that this new dentist would definitely not hurt me and that we should make an appointment right away.

On the drive home, my mom asked if I wanted straight teeth and would I be willing to go and meet this new dentist. She said his office was not very close to us, but she would drive me there to meet him and if I liked him, then she would find a way for me to get to my appointments.

Around this time, I had begun to notice how my smile was very different from my classmates so I didn't smile very much and actually tried to hide my teeth. I wanted to look better and be as pretty as the popular girls in school, especially those that got the main acting parts in the school plays. So, I agreed to try him out. In a few weeks we were off to meet this new dentist with the mysterious stuff called "laughing gas."

When we got to his office, I began to cry again uncontrollably and my hands shook so much that I could not even open the door. My mother told me it would be okay and opened the office door for us. I desperately wanted to run back to our car, but before I could act on that thought, a pretty, smiling lady came over to me, took my hand and led me into the reception room. She stopped at the front desk, pulled out two big square boxes from underneath the counter. When she opened them, I saw rings that were more beautiful than I could have ever imagined.

There were rings of all sizes, shapes and colors. They reminded me of some of the rings that I wanted from the gum ball machines, but could never seem to get, no matter how many times I put my money in.

As I gazed at this amazing box of jewels, she whispered in my ear that after each visit I could pick out any one that I wanted. I was mesmerized by this seemingly never ending row after row of pretty rings, that somehow I forgot my fear and my tears dried up. I felt a hand on my right shoulder and looked up and saw another smiling lady. She said she was the dentist's assistant and it was my turn to see him.

I was still thinking about which ring I wanted when I was done as she brought me into a room and asked me to jump into the chair so the dentist could do his examination.

I could feel myself beginning to fall apart, but she took my hand, told me her doctor was very nice, he would use the laughing gas and would not hurt me. I ready wanted to believe her.

I saw this man in a short, white coat entering the room and he introduced himself as Dr. P., the dentist. He had a kind face and was very good looking. He told me that he was just going to take some x-rays and look at my teeth and if I would let him, he would also fill some cavities.

He said he would use laughing gas and that it would help me relax and not be afraid and keep me from feeling any pain. I told him I did not want any needles. He took my hand and said, "Well, let's first see if you even have any cavities and then decide." For some reason, as afraid as I was, I felt I could trust him not to hurt me, so I said: "Okay."

After he did his exam, he told both my mother and me that I had a lot of cavities and it would take many appointments and suggested he fill some while I was there. I could already feel my tears pouring down my cheeks, but I let him put the mask on my nose while he instructed me to take deep breaths thru my nose and breath in the laughing gas. He told me to think of my favorite cartoon, which I did. As I thought of Alvin and the Chipmunks, I began to feel myself floating out of the chair and into another dimension far away from his office.

His assistant told me to open my mouth wide and she put some sweet jelly on my gums and had me bite on a stick. After a while, the dentist asked me if I felt tingly and like I was floating and when I said yes, his assistant held my hand and told me to open as wide as I could. I felt something long and metallic slide inside my mouth that felt like it was so long that it was traveling into space. Since it didn't really hurt, I did not care or react.

He told me I was doing well and to be very careful the rest of the day not to bite my cheek since my mouth was asleep and it would hurt later if I did. I could hear them talking and feel him working in my mouth. However, it was as if it was happening to someone else and not me. It was my first "out of body experience." Soon, I was told to rinse out my mouth and spit into a sink.

The mask was taken off of my nose and my lip and tongue felt thick and fat. I thought my face had grown. I was worried and asked if my lip was swollen and I was given a mirror and saw that my face looked exactly the same as before. It was pretty amazing. Nothing had hurt me.

The dentist took my hand and walked me to the reception area. He told my mother I had done very well and that I was numb and needed to be careful the rest of the day and not to bite myself. He also told me not to bite down hard for a few hours so the fillings could harden up and not fracture. Then, he told me that I could see his receptionist for a surprise.

While my mother made the next appointment, I stood staring at all the beautiful, shiny rings. I wanted all of them and could not decide. There were just too many choices. My mother was anxious to get home and prepare dinner. She told me to quickly choose one so we could leave. So, I picked the deep, ruby red one and put it on my finger and decided to pick a different one the next time.

This amazing, kind dentist with his smiling group of women and his magical "laughing gas" had won me over and totally changed my life. To this day I owe so very much to those wonderful people.

AUTHOR'S NOTE: In the summer of 2014, I decided to look up this wonderful dentist, Dr. P. to personally thank him for changing the path of my life. However, when I went online I found out that he had passed away the year before. Although I had sought him out before I made my final decision to go to dental school in 1976 and had gotten his blessing and encouragement then, I felt sad that I had missed my chance to really connect with him and let him know the full impact he had on my life.

BEYOND FEARFUL CHILD TO DENTAL SCHOOL

Well, dear readers, now you know how I went from fearful child to terrified pre-teenager to brave and willing "nitrousized" teenage dental patient.

Moving on, let me share with you how I chose dentistry as my career. In college, I chose the pre-medical career track wanting to be in a health service career involving biology. In my senior year I took an undergraduate research internship and enjoyed being mentored by a remarkable professor whom I admired. However, sacrificing animals for the sake of science and spending the entire day waiting for timers to go off so I could follow the next step became boring. More importantly, I missed the human contact since I was isolated in a lab most of the day.

I was seriously considering going to Veterinary school, but was unable to find a vet willing to allow me to shadow them to decide if that's what I wanted to do. There were no local veterinary schools and my parents urged me to stay close to home. I also knew financially it would be almost impossible.

As I was pondering exactly what I wanted to do, I met a female dentist who shared with me just how much she enjoyed her chosen field. As she described in detail what she did in an average day, the types of things she was able to do and the freedom of choices she had, I became intrigued. I told her about myself and my interests, and as I did so, I realized that dentistry might be an option for me. It was one that I never would have considered until I met her.

She told me that there were very few women in the field and getting accepted would be difficult and warned me that there would probably be many challenges along the way. However, she assured me that being a dentist would definitely be interesting and would fit my artistic, empathetic, caregiving and perfectionist nature.

I thought about it a lot and wondered if I could actually get into a career that had once terrified me and still made me anxious. I wondered if I could actually handle the kinds of patients like I used to be and still would be if I hadn't been given the nitrous oxide (laughing gas).

I decided to meet with my dentist, Dr. P., and get his opinion and ask more specific questions about what he did and what he liked about being a dentist.

I called him up and made an appointment. When I went to his office, he told me that he was quite surprised in my interest, but very willing to discuss and share what he knew. He was extremely encouraging and told me that I could do a lot of good knowing what I personally knew about dental fear. He also intimated that being a woman and having smaller hands than a man's, would make it easier working in the mouth and treating patients.

I left his office encouraged, yet still unsure, but now I was definitely considering the possibility of going to dental school. As I was considering what I should do next and feeling pressured to make some decision, I decided to take a year off after graduation to work and save some money and to give myself more time to decide exactly what I wanted to do. I thought it would help me if I could get some actual hands on knowledge at a dental clinic. So, I applied and was accepted for a volunteer dental assistant position at the Cleft Palate Institute at Tufts University Dental School. I was more than a little concerned about just how I would handle being in a dental environment all day. I wondered if my dental anxiety would return and limit me or if I would enjoy it when it wasn't me in the chair. I knew that would be the ultimate test and would help me make my final decision.

To my utter amazement, I was absolutely fascinated by everything. All of the dentists and their staffs were nice and allowed me to watch and observe all the procedures performed. After some time had passed, I was even allowed to step in and suction and hand various instruments to the dentists as they were treating their patients. It was incredibly interesting to me and eventually I could feel myself wanting to just jump in and be the dentist. I learned a lot of useful information. However, the best part of the experience for me was that I realized that I had no dental anxiety at all. At that point I also realized that I could actually enjoy being a dentist.

So, I got the applications for the dental schools that interested me, took the remaining required pre-requisite courses and sent off my applications with hopes that I would be granted an interview by at least one of them.

I had been warned by many of the people at the clinic that there were many applicants and not many spaces available. They told me that it was very competitive and that very few women had ever been accepted. They encouraged me to apply, but warned me not to get my hopes up and to remember that rejections are the rule not the exception.

AUTHOR'S NOTE: When I started dental school in June of 1977, there were very few women enrolled in dental schools across the United States. I was told it was less than 5% when I was accepted. Then, there was a change of sentiment in the dental community which led to an increase in the number of women in the profession. So, in 1978, female first year dental students comprised 15.9%, according to the ADA Health Policy Institute unpublished 2014 findings from the Survey of Dental Practice. (ADA News January 18, 2016, pages 1, 14) Since 1978, there has been a continuous rise in the number of women applying to and being accepted into dental school.

> **This increase rose to 43.5% in 2003-2004 and then jumped to 46.7% in the 2013-2014 academic years. (Taken from the ADA Health Policy Institute, hpi@ada.org)**

Well, as worried as that made me, I was not going to be a quitter. I had finally found something that I wanted to do and believed that I could be quite good at and even help a lot of people along the way. So, I prayed and waited.

I was granted a few interviews. When I went to my first one at Tufts, I was told to sit and wait with the other dozen applicants. As I sat there, I began to feel less confident and more anxious as the minutes ticked by. I listened to many of them chatter away about all their accomplishments and their excellent GPA's (grade point averages). All I could do was to stay calm and ignore what the others were saying and try not to compare myself to them.

When they called my name, I shook the interviewer's hand and in my nervous state took a seat on the nice comfortable desk chair. Well, when I saw his surprised reaction, I realized that I was now seated in the dean's chair. I will not bore you with all the details and will only say that we both had a laugh over my faux pas and it turned into a very good interview.

So much so, that I received my acceptance letter a few months later. I immediately sent in my acceptance response and fee to hold my spot to start Tufts Dental School the next semester.

There is no need to go into the grueling next four years. However, I must say that I found out that I "loved" treating patients in the clinic. I also enjoyed helping the frightened children stay calm and ultimately get their dental care done.

As an undergraduate we learned how to use nitrous oxide (laughing gas), and even had one class on hypnosis, but we were usually not allowed to do any of it until we were graduates working in the post-graduate clinic. Therefore, when we students worked on one another, I had to get over my dental fear completely in order to fully participate in my class and fulfill my requirements.

I remember thinking how grateful I was to Dr. P., and how he had helped me get to this phase of my life.

When I graduated, I took lots of continuing education courses to improve my clinical and personal skills. It also required some participation (hands on) classes on using "nitrous oxide" and other pain free techniques. I not only wanted to be an excellent dentist, but I also wanted to especially help those people that were like me (or should I say the way that I "had" been).

When I started my first practice in Boise, Idaho, I was one of the first two women dentists who passed the Idaho Dental Boards. Many patients said that they came to see me because I was a woman. I was told many times that they believed a woman would be more gentle, more caring, more understanding and that our smaller hands would create less pain for them.

OBTAINING CLINICAL SKILLS, HELPING PATIENTS AND BECOMING AN ANTI-ANXIETY ADVOCATE

Discovering Techniques and Seeing Fearful Patients Respond

In my first two years practicing, I was constantly amazed just how many patients had dental anxiety and how many requested the nitrous oxide that I had intentionally installed in my operatories, the rooms where dentists treat their patients.

I was told in dental school that many people had dental fear and, as a result, did not go to a dentist. But, I was not really prepared to find so many patients that reminded me of where I came from. I had expected to meet a few fearful patients and was thrilled that I was able to help them. Interestingly enough, as the word spread that I had nitrous oxide available and that I had a gentle and painless way of treating people, more and more of these patients came my way.

I soon discovered that using nitrous oxide and my gentle techniques were not always enough. I began to meet more and more adults outside of my office environment that had not been to any dentist for many years, sometimes over thirty years and many from early childhood. The majority of them either inferred or outright told me of their fear of dentists. I began to hear outrageous stories of dental pain, trauma and even abuse at the hands of a dental professional. Boy, were my eyes opened. It brought back my own terrifying memories and awful dental experiences that I had attributed to having an unsympathetic dentist.

Some of the stories I was told were of dentists not using anesthetic, telling the patient that they did not need any or that baby teeth don't hurt so no anesthetic was needed. Others involved patients being told that they were numb when they were not, being berated, yelled at and being made to feel intimidated. There were even some stories of actual abuse. I learned more than I ever really expected or wanted to know.

Since I had been one of those terrified patients at one time, I made a very conscious decision that I would be extremely gentle and caring, use nitrous oxide and dedicate myself to finding any and all ways to help as many anxious and fearful people as I could. I felt these patients needed somewhere to go where they felt safe and taken care of. I knew that there were very few options available at that time. My original goal was to emulate my savior dentist and follow in his footsteps, but I felt a strong need to even go one step further.

It was a confirmation and validation to me when many of my new patients indicated that they had been referred by a friend who had told them I treated all fearful patients with empathy and respect and took great care to make their appointments as painless as possible.

As time went on and I expanded my clinical skills in giving anesthetic in a painless manner, (the "dreaded shot"), I attended courses in patient management, treating fear and helping patients emotionally as well as psychologically.

I also attended continuing education courses in Acupressure, Hypnosis, NLP (Neuro-Linguistic Programming) and eventually in Non-IV Oral Conscious Sedation.

Becoming an Anti-Anxiety Advocate

I have always found it interesting and somewhat amazing when I meet someone who tells me that they chose their career when they were a child. They also shared that they just "knew" what they wanted to be "when they grew up."

I have heard stories of people who had taken in animals and nursed them back to health. Because of the experience, they wanted to become a veterinarian and spend their lives saving animals. Some have shared with me their plans to become doctors, nurses, firemen, architects, accountants, policemen, actors, pilots, and the list goes on. Their choses were based on their early childhood experiences. Some had parents or family members as role models to help choose professions. However, many did not.

I always knew that I wanted to make a difference in the world and since I loved animals, I had thought of becoming a veterinarian.

However, never in my wildest dreams would I have thought that my greatest fear, that of going to a dentist, would ultimately lead me to my "spiritual calling" of becoming a dentist specializing in treating patients with fear and anxiety of the dental chair. It was quite a surprise to me and a real extraordinary journey when I overcame my fear of dentists and realized that I could take my own personal experiences and make a difference in other people's lives.

It was a welcome revelation the day that I realized that I could use my gift and skills to actually help dental phobics overcome their fears, improve their self-esteem and gain a sense of control.

How could I deny others of this gift and why would I even want to. My future no longer looked blank and filled with the unknown. It actually felt like the choice had been made for me by some higher order in the universe.

I became not only excited by the prospect, but I also developed a powerful passion to help people change their lives for the better. Thus, I began my search for the best techniques and tools to change people's dental experiences from those of fear, panic and psychic pain to those of comfort, safety, peacefulness and calmness.

My mission of being an anti-anxiety advocate was born and has stayed strong within me. I feel the dental profession has come very far since my early days, but there is still a long way for it to go.

So, I invite you to use whatever you find helpful in this book and to offer it to anyone you think could benefit.

How This Book Can Help You

This book is a *Dental Guide* written to answer questions you have about dental anxiety. It is designed to offer you options currently available and a "road map" for finding them. This book allows those with dental anxiety to identify their specific fears and to feel understood, validated and hopeful that they can do something about it.

It offers confirmation that you are not alone and that there are dentists that understand and care about what you go through and want to help you overcome whatever has blocked you. The many personal stories shared in this book can offer you renewed hope and inspiration. By learning how others have overcome their dental fear can give you confidence that you too can be relieved of your fear of the dental chair.

Additionally, you will find a multitude of suggestions and possibilities that you may have been unaware of that can help minimize and alleviate the fears that are stopping you from going to the dentist. I believe that the sections on NLP or Neuro-Linguistic Programming provide an insightful introduction to this amazing life changing process. The stories are "real world" and revealing experiences of some of my patients. They show how you too can change your personal experiences during your next dental visit.

This book will enlighten all readers on the "reality" of dental anxiety and highlights dental terms and definitions that some of you may have heard of but never quite understood. The goal is to help explain the essence of the fear that you, your friends and/or your loved ones may have regarding dental anxiety and to empower you to be proactive and ask specific questions of your dentist and other dental professionals.

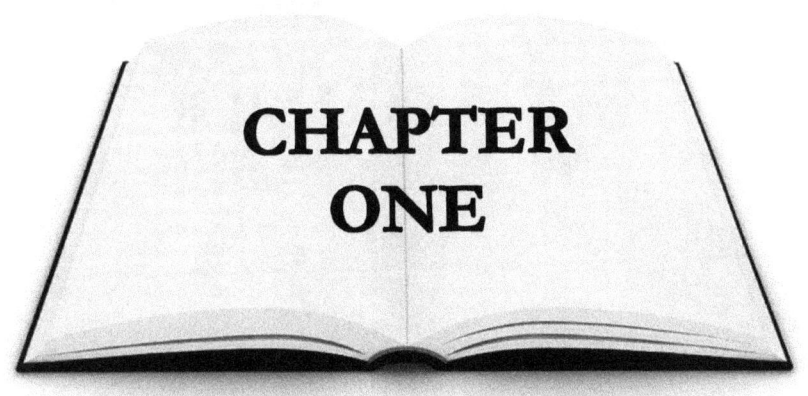

UNDERSTANDING DENTAL FEAR AND COMMON FEARS OF A DENTAL PATIENT

What is the Dental Profession Saying?

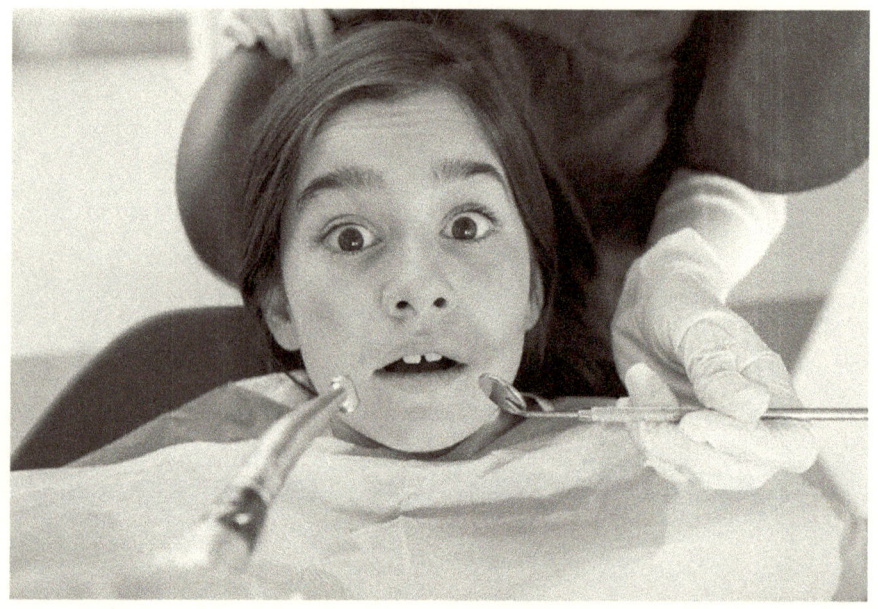

"Dentists reported more relaxed patients, among younger people, whose first dental experience is for prevention and not for decay treatment."

ACCORDING TO THE DENTAL PROFESSION

According to the American Dental Association (ADA) in April 1999, there were an estimated 35 million adults that experience dental anxiety. According to the article "Controlling Pain and Anxiety" (by Caroline Bouffard, written in Access, April 1999), "These dental fears can stem from past experiences, popular films and television sitcoms, and domestic or sexual abuse." She goes on to say that dental procedures can be "associated with the loss of control" and the dental team may appear as a "hostile entity with the power to inflict pain and pass judgment."

She explains that the majority of these anxious patients have had a traumatic dental visit in the past. In the article, she states the following, "They have had a dentist whom they felt didn't give them enough anesthetic, scared them, belittled them for not tolerating the procedure, rushed them into things, or didn't answer questions."

Then, in May of 2002, an article was written in the AGD Impact magazine saying that "dental anxiety is easing up." The article states: "Dentists reported more relaxed patients, among younger people, whose first dental experience is for prevention and not for decay treatment. In addition, dentists themselves are doing a better job of easing anxieties by taking a more humane approach by being concerned about the person's feelings." (AGD Impact Magazine, May 2002)

However in that same magazine, Dr Arthur A. Weiner, a professor, researcher and author of behavioral dentistry says that "many still don't seek dental care due to *painful past experiences* or even inaccurate representations of dental experiences on television and in the movies." He then goes on to say that "there are about 25 million Americans who don't go to the dentist because of fear and anxiety."

WHAT MY RESEARCH REVEALED

My research has shown that it used to be over 50% of the population that did not seek dental care because of their dental anxiety. Fortunately the number is decreasing, since most of the current articles, as of 2014, say that it is now closer to 40%.

Interestingly enough a recent figure taken from the Journal of the American Dental Association, (JADA, 146 (8), August 2015, Pg 642) showed that 33.9 million people visit a physician and do not have private Dental Benefits and do not visit a dentist.

A question I am constantly asked is, "What are the typical fears of a dental patient?" From my perspective, there is no "typical" fear, but many of my patient's fears have aspects of one or a combination of more than one kind. The next section contains a list of the types of fears that I have seen in my practice. I believe that I have listed most of the common fears. However, being human, I may have missed your specific situation. If that is the case, please e-mail me or send me your story by contacting me at fatnomorebook@gmail.com or via my website at www.susanrcushing.com.

COMMON FEARS OF A DENTAL PATIENT

I believe every one of these fears come from an originating incident. A person may not remember it, may be blocking it out, may be totally unaware of the source of the fear, may be in denial of where it came from, may not want to remember it, for some reason, or may have something that makes them fearful buried deep inside.

I also believe in "body memories" and that when we are traumatized or assaulted in some way at some time in our lives, our neurons (nerves) remember it and store the information inside our bodies. Then, if we are placed in a situation that our neurons remember as resembling that traumatic event and how painful it was, our protective consciousness uses fear to keep us from replicating the event.

Based on my research, here is a list of the most common fears of a dental patient:

- ✓ Generalized, unspecific fear with no specific reason attached, (at least none that a person can remember).
- ✓ Specific fear, well defined and remembered. This could include being hurt by a dental professional, hearing someone's painful scream while in an operatory or smelling a terrible odor at a dental office, such as burning teeth, medicines or blood. The fear could arise from other experiences such as being tied down in a papoose board as a child or being restricted in some way during an appointment and feeling vulnerable or unsafe. The list goes on.
- ✓ Fear of needles (also called needle phobia).
- ✓ Fear of being in pain and of being hurt. This can happen in a variety of ways and includes fear coming from a prior bad experience being repeated. A survey done by the ADA Survey Center in 1997 wrote that "Fear of pain is the greatest factor keeping people from visiting their dentist." The survey showed that 60% would be more likely to visit the dentist if they did not have this fear of

the pain. (ADA Survey Center, 1997, Survey of Consumer Attitudes and Behavior Regarding Dental Issues).

- ✓ Fear of gagging or choking.
- ✓ Fear of being powerless, vulnerable or being seen as vulnerable.
- ✓ Fear of being victimized or abused (This may be related to past dental abuse or childhood sexual abuse issues).
- ✓ Fear of being unable to breathe.
- ✓ Fear of being asphyxiated or suffocated, usually related to a prior incident, possibly with a nitrous oxide mask or some other event.
- ✓ Fear of "Lock Jaw" or one's mouth being unable to close. This may be from a past experience of a person's jaw locking when open too wide, prior TMJD ((Temporomandibular Joint Dysfunction) issues or pain when opening too wide and fear the joint might lock.
- ✓ Fear of lying down fully flat in a dental chair. This can be related to fear of feeling vulnerable, possibly from having the condition of vertigo, back issues, medical issues or from some past unsafe incident.
- ✓ Fear of the drill or the sound of drilling. This can be the sound itself hurting one's ears, bringing back a painful memory or one's imagining the drill in their mouth as "bigger than life."
- ✓ Fear of being berated, laughed at or mocked.
- ✓ Fear of being embarrassed or feeling stupid.
- ✓ Fear of the unknown. This might be related to their dental findings or what treatment will be needed.

- ✓ Fear of the known. Once a person knows what dental problems they have, then they feel they have to deal with it emotionally in some way.
- ✓ Fear of the anesthetic or any anesthesia.
- ✓ Fear of dying.
- ✓ Fear of being numb and what it is doing to them physically and emotionally.
- ✓ Fear of someone else seeing and knowing what is inside their mouth. This is also a fear of being *"exposed."* The mouth is a very personal space and some people feel it is their secret just how they care for themselves and that it will be discovered.
- ✓ Fear of Judgment and what others will think of them. This might include feeling shame of their level of fear or of their personal dental status.
- ✓ Fear of the cost and being unable to afford to get treatment and feeling bad about it.
- ✓ Fear of just being touched.
- ✓ Fear of anyone getting close to them, intrusion of one's personal space, especially their mouth and face.
- ✓ Fear of disapproval or not being accepted.
- ✓ Fear of being unable to communicate personal needs while "under the dentist's control."
- ✓ Fear of being left alone in the room.
- ✓ Fear of being pressured to do something and being unable to say "no." This includes fear of being taken advantage of or talked into something they do not want and being unable to be assertive and stand up for themselves.

- ✓ Fear of screaming, crying, getting out of control and perhaps even biting the dentist.
- ✓ Fear of their beliefs, desires, wishes or requests being compromised.
- ✓ Fear of closing their eyes or the fear of getting something in their eyes.
- ✓ Fear of "catching" some disease at the office and the lack of infection control.

  > I have found that many patients have hidden fears about being contaminated or "catching" something at the dental office. Let me reassure you that infection control is highly regulated and dental offices work hard to comply. It is easy to verify this either by asking when you call or checking it out at your appointment to see if all the instruments used are "bagged, tagged and sterilized" for each patient.

- ✓ Fear of loss of control. In an article from Access, April 1999, page 17, it says, "The feeling of control can disappear the moment a member of the oral health care team does something that the patient is not expecting or does not understand. So, it is important to explain each procedure at each appointment."
- ✓ Fear of hospitals or clinics.
- ✓ Fear of white coats, called "white coat syndrome."
- ✓ Fear of "root canals" or other specific procedures.
- ✓ Fear of paresthesia or becoming paralyzed for life.
- ✓ Fear of being a "chicken" or wimpy and being seen as "different."

- ✓ Fear of not knowing or understanding what will be done to them or for them, including exposing their lack of dental knowledge.

- ✓ Fear of getting cold sores and/or any post-operative consequences from any dental procedure.

- ✓ Fear of any foreign body being placed inside their mouth, including the actual instruments or any filling materials.

- ✓ Fear of not getting fully anesthetized no matter how much anesthetic is given. This usually is a result of having past dental treatment and not being fully numb while the dentist continued treatment anyway, causing great pain to the patient.

- ✓ Fear of the vibration of the drill and possibly needing to move and having the drill cut them. This can be either the actual feeling of the drill vibrating or fear of being damaged irreparably from the drill.

- ✓ Fear of swallowing something foreign.

> Recently, I had a Non-IV Oral Conscious Sedation patient have difficulty during a procedure and she kept clutching at her throat. Her throat was fully protected by a device we use called an Isolite. I verified that her throat was clear and reassured her there was nothing in her throat. I gave her time to swallow on her own, but she kept doing the same behavior. I felt sure that she was safe and she told me to proceed, but I knew there was something else going on that we had not addressed. The next day, when I spoke with her, she told me that she was glad that I had done as she requested and completed all her work. She also said that she had figured out what happened. She shared with me that she had a memory from thirteen years ago of her dearest friend dying of

cancer. Her friend's lungs kept filling up with fluid and she was choking to death. Ever since then, she has had this fear of choking to death herself that she was not consciously aware of. It was pretty fresh in her unconscious though, because ironically her beloved pet was going through the same issue. I also have seen this fear as a direct result of child abuse memories.

- ✓ Fear of getting one's hopes up and then being rejected and turned away because their mouth is so bad, it cannot be repaired.

- ✓ Fear and intimidation by authority figures at a dental office. (This may also include hearing horror stories from others and imagining the worst)

- ✓ Fear of what kind of dental materials the office uses. Some patients are very concerned about what is "hidden" in the filling materials used, specifically what is in the silver fillings (amalgam). They worry that the mercury used to make it will be released into their bodies as a toxin.

There have been many studies done on the safety of amalgam fillings. In 2009, the U.S. Food and Drug Administration evaluated the research and found no reason to limit the use of amalgam, saying it was safe for adults and children over six years of age (U.S. Food and Drug Administration, Appendix I, July 28, 2009).

However, there are some groups that are not convinced and feel they have seen some harmful side effects and detrimental medical consequences as a direct result of the amalgam in patient's mouths. They asked the FDA to reconsider and that review is still under way.

If you are concerned and do not want any silver fillings or amalgams placed in your mouth, preferring white or composite (plastic) fillings, then it is up to you to be proactive. Always remember that patients have the choice of what material gets placed in their mouths. I suggest that you research the potential dental office beforehand or interview the dentist "before" starting any dental work. Let the dentist know that you do not want any kind of silver fillings (amalgam) placed in your teeth.

In a recent article published by the American Association of Endodontists (AAE) in their winter 2015 newsletter the following was written: "According to a February 2015 AAE online survey, root canal treatment is the dental procedure that makes Americans most apprehensive. Fifty-six percent said root canal treatment would cause anxiety, followed by tooth extraction (47%) and placement of a dental implant (42%). Women are more likely than men to say dental procedures make them anxious, including root canal treatment (62% vs. 48%), tooth extraction (54% vs. 39%) and dental implant placement (49% vs. 35%). However, a 2008 AAE consumer awareness survey found that patients who have experienced root canal treatment are six times more likely to describe it as *painless* than patients who have not had root canal treatment."

When one considers all the possible fears associated with a dental appointment, you can see that it takes a huge amount of courage for many people to not only come to the dentist but also to just open up their mouths once they are there.

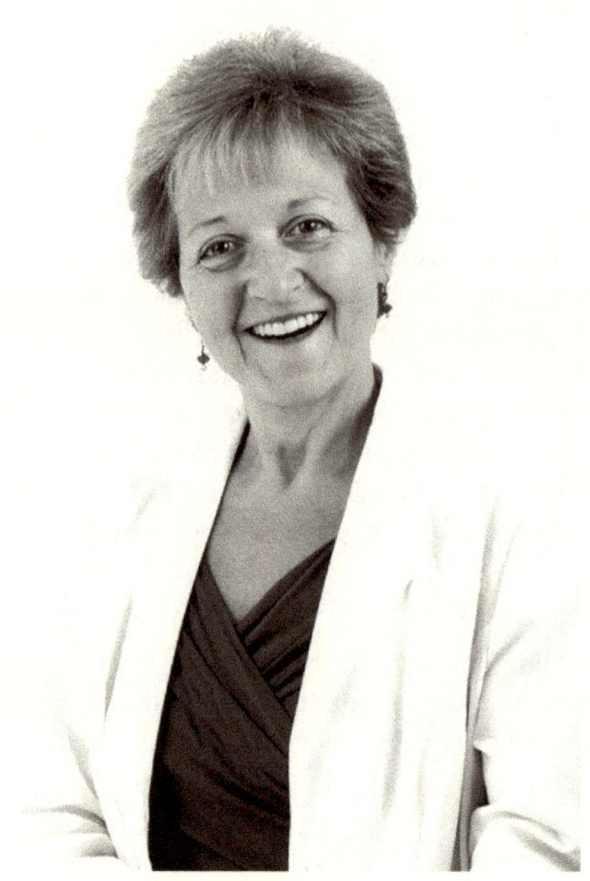

"I feel rather strongly that no one should be expected to endure pain during their dental treatment."

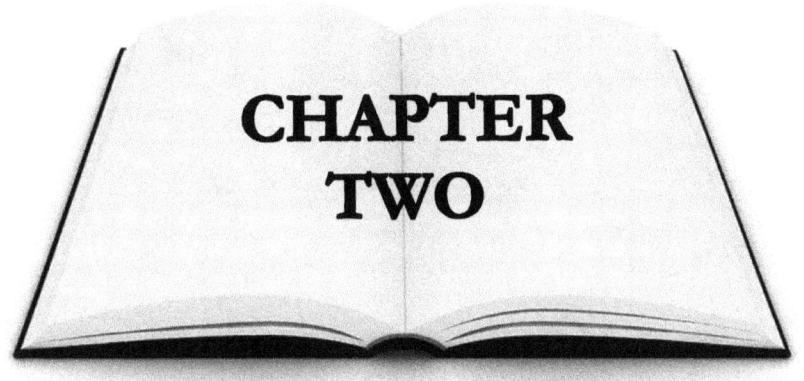

CHAPTER TWO

COMMON ANESTHETICS AND PAIN PREVENTION

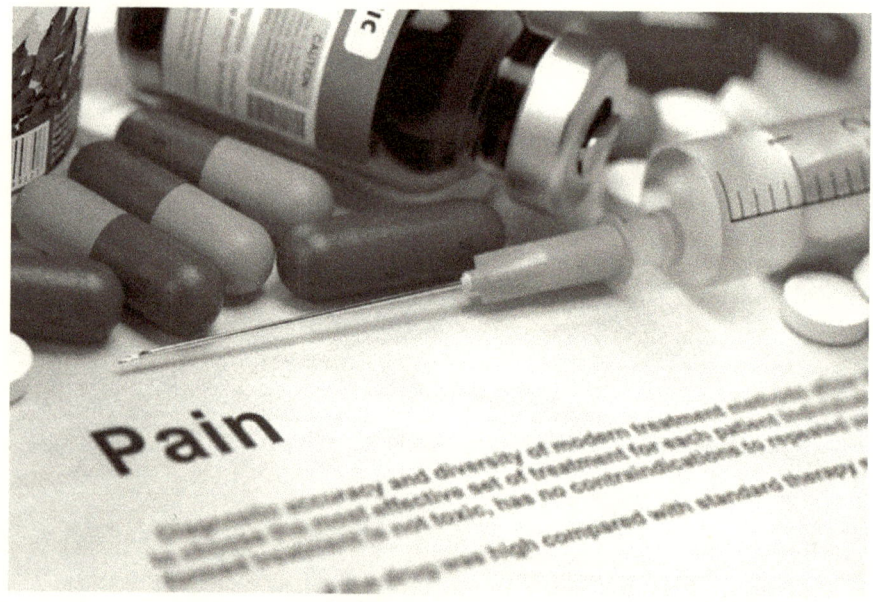

"In medicine pain relates to a sensation that hurts. If you feel pain it hurts. You could feel discomfort, distress or anxiety depending on the severity and your individual perception of it."

LOCAL ANESTHETICS

In dentistry, local anesthetics are used for the temporary loss of sensation or pain in a part of the mouth allowing the dentist to do what is necessary during their patient's treatment. The anesthetic is either topically applied or injected and does not depress the patient's level of consciousness.

The dentist chooses a particular anesthetic, depending on the area of the mouth being treated, the patient's specific medical issues, the time planned for the treatment and the time needed for the anesthetic to take effect. For example, a patient with a cardiac or heart condition may warrant an anesthetic with less stress on the heart and a child needs an anesthetic that takes affect rather quickly and wears off quickly, so they have less time to injure themselves after the appointment, due to the numbness.

I feel rather strongly that "no one" should be expected to endure pain during their dental treatment.

In preparing for a patient's dental treatment, most dentists will apply a topical anesthetic directly onto the area to be injected. This topical is used to alleviate the pain from the needle as it enters the tissue. These products contain drugs such as Benzocaine, Lidocaine and Tetracaine.

Patients can also purchase various topical anesthetics over the counter and use them to minimize the pain from teething, canker sores, braces and even toothaches. Most of these topical anesthetics contain the same medications that you get in the injection, but are stronger in order to permeate the tissue.

When a dentist needs to numb an area of the mouth, the anesthetic is injected into the gum or cheek trying to get as close as possible to the location of the nerve responsible for numbing the teeth being treated. The most common anesthetic used is

Lidocaine, although a newer one called *Articaine* is gaining quite a bit of popularity, due to its ability to permeate the tissues in the area more effectively.

This numbing part is only one ingredient of what is actually injected. The liquid can also include the following:

(1) a drug called a *vasoconstrictor* which narrows the blood vessels making the numbness last longer;

(2) a chemical that keeps the vasoconstrictor from breaking down;

(3) *Sodium Chloride* that helps the drug get into the bloodstream; and

(4) *Sodium Hydroxide* that helps the numbing agent work.

Occasionally, a patient will have an adverse reaction to one of these additives and will need a different anesthetic made for that specific purpose. These local anesthetics can last for several hours, so it's important for patients to be extremely careful after their dental treatment and not bite down or play with the numb area whereby injuring themselves.

Although these local anesthetics are the common drugs used in the dental office, there are some side effects that patients must be aware of. Although rare, a patient must know they exist and understand the possibility of their occurrence.

One possible side effect is where the needle can enter a nerve during the injection process and injure it. If a nerve should be damaged in this way a patient might have numbness and associated pain for several weeks or months. However, the nerve will usually heal with time.

Another side effect is when the medicine causes numbness outside of the intended area. This may result in a patient's eyelid or mouth drooping. When the anesthetic wears off, the numbness and drooping are gone. Also a patient may notice that they cannot blink. This usually only lasts a few hours and is back to normal when the anesthetic wears off.

The anesthetic can cause a *hematoma*, which is a blood-filled swelling. It happens when the needle hits a blood vessel. When the blood leaves the occupied space, the hematoma is gone.

Lastly, the vasoconstrictor drug in the liquid injected can cause the heart to beat faster. This almost always lasts only a minute or so and is what many patients incorrectly think of as an allergic reaction.

Allergic reactions to our modern day anesthetics are quite rare. However, it is of utmost importance that a patient tells the dentist about all the medication they are taking, even if they do not think it is important.

Other ways to control the sensation and perception of pain at a dental office is with the use of "laughing gas" or *nitrous oxide*. Nitrous oxide reduces one's stress and allows better pain control within the body and with sedation.

Sedation includes oral conscious sedation, where a patient is put in a state between consciousness and unconsciousness, but can still respond if needed and General Anesthesia, where a patient is fully unconscious and being controlled by the use of IV drugs and monitored closely by an anesthesiologist.

From my perspective, once patients find a dentist they like, trust and feel safe with, they should be able to trust that dentist with choosing the most effective anesthetic for their benefit according to the procedure being done.

It is a patient's responsibility to inform the dentist beforehand if they have any allergies, anesthetic reactions, drug preferences and concerns, medical issues, medication currently being taken and any concerns about being numb.

However, once all that is done, I feel it is up to the treating dentist's knowledge and skill to choose what anesthetic should be used, including the specific anesthetic, whether it is a short-acting or a long-acting one or if specific anesthetic protocol is required that would be in the best interest of that patient.

As in any medical situation, once you have done all your research, choosing who you want to treat you, deciding on the treatment to be done and giving informed consent, it is important to allow that medical practitioner to do what they believe is best for your particular problem.

Here is a list of the most common anesthetics used in modern dentistry.

Novocaine

Novocaine is the most common term that patients use when asking about anesthetics for their dental treatment. However, since I have been practicing dentistry (1981) it is no longer used.

Articaine or Septocaine

Articaine or Septocaine is a very effective and moderate lasting anesthetic that has become extremely popular.

Lidocaine HCL or Xylocaine

Lidocaine HCL or Xylocaine (with or without epinephrine) is commonly used to anesthetize both upper and lower teeth. It is most effective when a dentist is giving a lower mandibular block, to fully anesthetize an entire half of the lower arch. The epinephrine keeps the anesthetic localized around the injection area allowing a more profound or stronger anesthesia.

Mepivacaine HCL (Carbocaine) or Polocaine

Mepivacaine HCL (Carbocaine) or Polocaine, that has no epinephrine, are commonly used for short procedures in adults and children, in order to limit the amount of time being numb. It is recommended as a safe and effective anesthetic for people with heart conditions and is also advised when a patient has a sensitivity "reaction" when exogenous epinephrine is introduced into their body.

Marcaine

Marcaine is a very, very long acting anesthetic that is used most often for lower extractions and when doing mandibular quadrant dentistry (restoring an entire half arch of lower teeth).

Prilocaine HCL or Citanest Forte with epinephrine

Prilocaine HCL or Citanest Forte with epinephrine is used for rapid onset and is free of the preservative methylparaben that can cause an adverse reaction in some patients.

Prilocaine HCL or Citanest Plain without epinephrine is for rapid onset and is free of methylparaben.

TOPICAL Anesthetics

TOPICAL Anesthetics can be in many forms including ointments, liquid or spray. The most common used in dentistry are made with either Benzocaine or Lidocaine. It is very important to note that Topical Anesthetic, used to pre-anesthetize the tissue prior to the injection is a very effective way to minimize the sting of "the shot."

I feel strongly that it should be placed before any injection is given, unless a patient is allergic, of course. It also helps if a patient takes two ibuprofen (i.e. Advil) and two acetaminophen (i.e. Tylenol) prior to any major dental procedure. This helps minimize their discomfort during and after treatment.

PAIN PREVENTION

In dentistry, pain relates to a sensation that physically hurts. If you feel pain, it hurts. That pain might cause you to feel various levels of discomfort, distress or anxiety depending on its severity and your individual perception of it. Your pain might be steady and constant and feel like a dull ache, it may be pulsating and throbbing or it could be pinching or stabbing. Your pain could come and go or it could linger for minutes to hours. It could be set off upon eating or from hot or cold foods. Each type of pain helps the dentist determine the origin of it, the most likely diagnosis and ways to treat the patient to eliminate the pain and correct the problem.

Of course the ideal way to treat a patient's pain is to find the source and treat it immediately. However, that is not always possible. Also, after dental work is accomplished a patient may have post-operative pain that will need pain relief.

Pain Management with the Use of Nonopioid and Opioid Analgesics

Aspirin and ibuprofen belong to a large class of drugs known as nonsteroidal anti-inflammatory drugs, commonly called NSAIDs. NSAIDs, like Advil, Aleve and Motrin, and acetaminophen (Tylenol), can block pain and reduce fever. Together, they make up the most widely used group of drugs for treating pain conditions.

The most common non-opioid analgesics used in a dental office are acetaminophen and NSAIDs.

Most cases of postoperative pain include an inflammatory component. For this reason NSAIDs are the most rational first-line agents and are often superior to conventional dosages of opioids.

Aspirin may also be used for dental pain but as an analgesic and antipyretic (reducing fever) acetaminophen is equal in potency and effectiveness to aspirin. Aspirin reduces fever and lessens swelling and is advised for mild to moderate pain. It can also be used in the treatment of inflammation, but that is not its main purpose.

However for more severe pain most dentists will advise NSAIDs or an aspirin-narcotic combination.

Since all drugs have side effects, it is very important that a patient inform their dentist (or doctor) about any allergies or reactions they have to a prescribed medication.

From my thirty-five years of experience, if a patient is undergoing major dental treatment that includes many teeth, a large section of the mouth, a long appointment or will be keeping their mouth open for an extended period of time, they should take a combination of acetaminophen and NSAIDs prior to their dental treatment. Of course, this is as long as they have no known medical contraindications with these drugs.

This combination will help minimize any post-operative pain, soreness or inflammation. I have followed this regimen for many years and it has worked well keeping my patients comfortable and usually pain free.

What I suggest for any anxious patient I am treating is to consider trying "laughing gas." It will decrease any pain you might experience during your treatment, allow your anesthetics to work more effectively and it will give you a completely different dental experience and change your perspective and paradigm regarding going to the dentist.

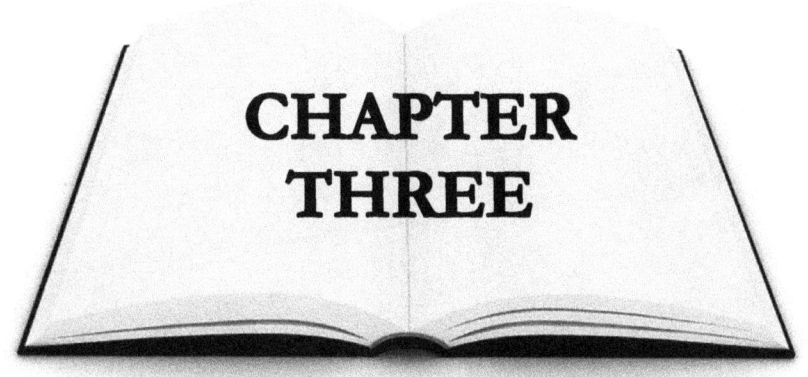

CHAPTER THREE

THE REASONS PATIENTS SCHEDULE APPOINTMENTS

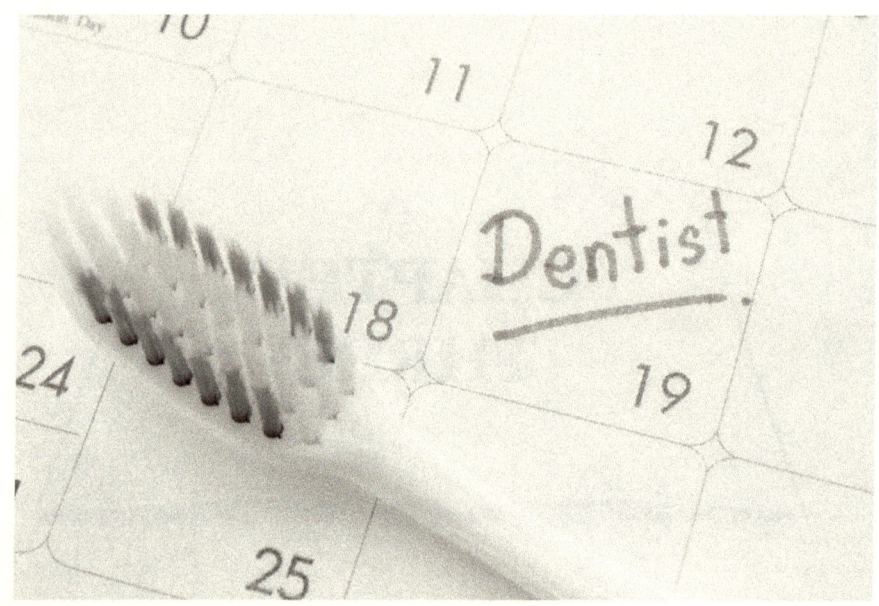

"Very phobic patients might schedule a consult only, in order to interview the dental team, especially the dentist before allowing anyone to look into their mouths."

Many fearful patients will call to schedule a cleaning appointment as their way to meet the dentist and staff and decide if they like them and can trust them. Very phobic patients might schedule a consult only, in order to interview the dental team, especially the dentist before allowing anyone to look into their mouths. Many of these patients are even anxious about getting their teeth cleaned.

The most common reasons that patients schedule appointments are:

(1) Pain or infection-both of these are great motivators;

(2) Wanting a cleaning;

(3) Having a specific area of concern as a broken tooth or swollen gum, or wanting a few teeth looked at BEFORE any pain develops;

(4) Wanting a complete exam or "check-up"; and

(5) Any combination of the four reasons above.

It never ceases to amaze me how a potential patient will check out the hygienist first and if they like them and can trust them, they will open up and ask questions about the dentist. If they like what they hear, then they are more comfortable scheduling an appointment with the dentist.

HAVE NO FEAR OF THE DENTAL CHAIR!

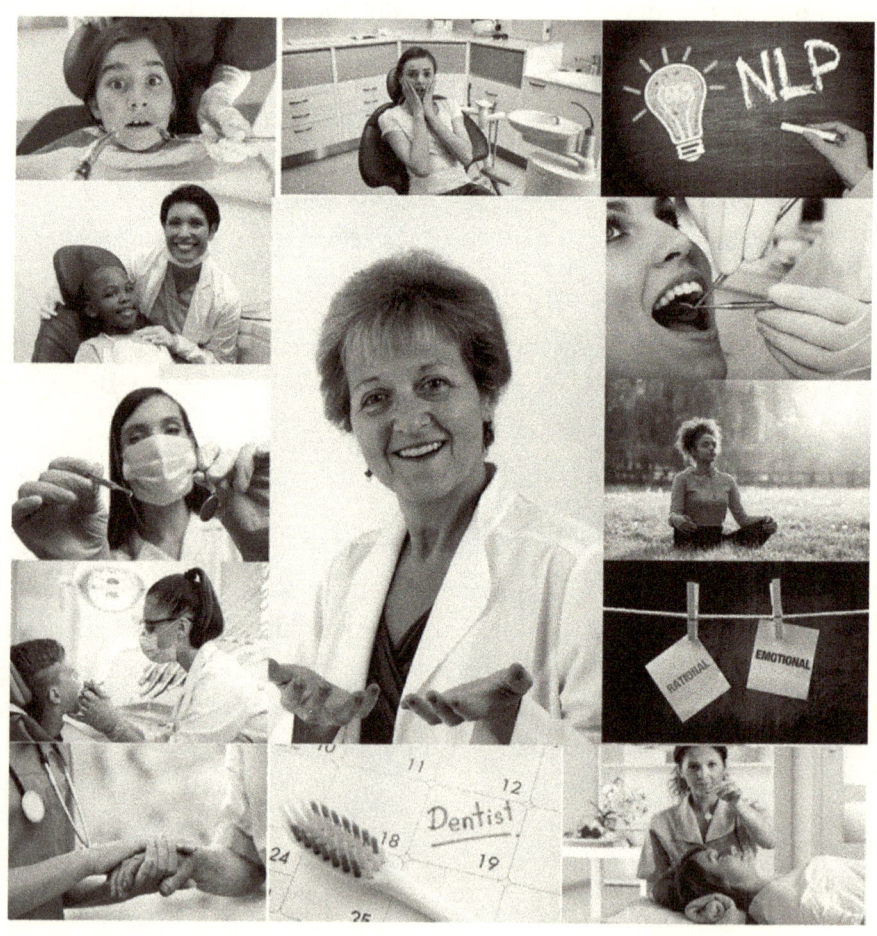

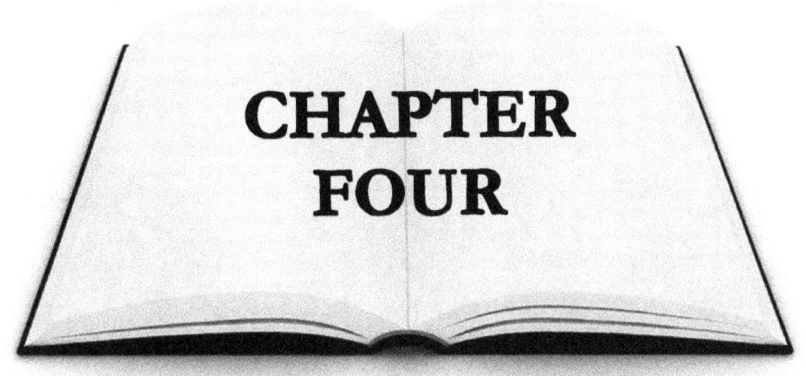

CHAPTER FOUR

ANXIETY REDUCING TOOLS

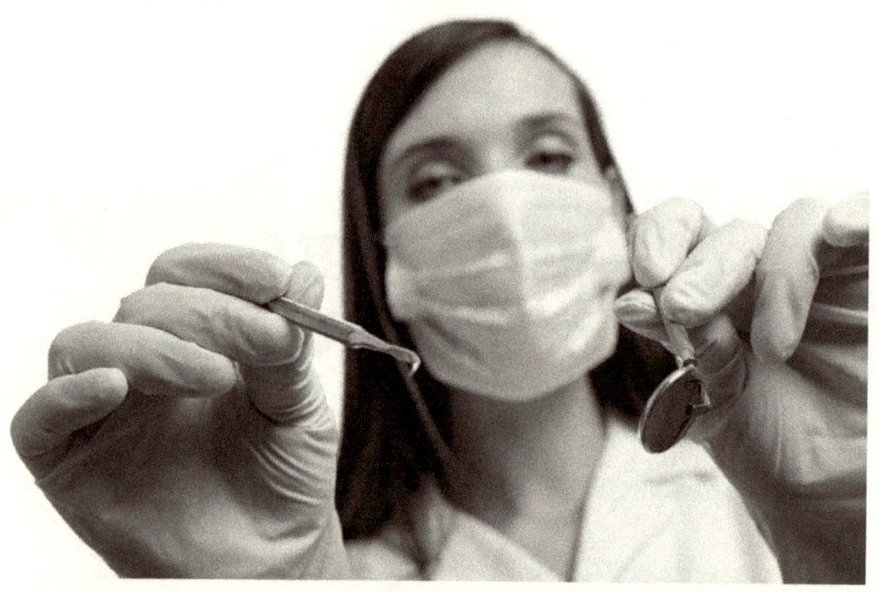

"All dentists have their own arsenal of tools to help a patient reduce and manage their dental anxiety. Some are what I would call common sense."

All dentist have their own arsenal of tools to help a patient reduce and manage their dental anxiety. Some are what I would call "common sense." Some come naturally to most dentists, some require spending additional time with the patient, some require additional training and then practice, and some come from pure experience with trial and error along the way.

From what I have seen the most effective tools are the result of empathy and being truly able to experience things as if you were in the patient's shoes. For me, this came from "living it." For many it comes from taking the time to imagine and be open to a patient's reality.

THE TEN BEST TOOLS FOR REDUCING ANXIETY

1. A very effective tool is for a dentist to go into the reception room themselves, greet their patient with a warm, pleasant welcoming smile, hold out a hand and guide their patient to the treatment room. It is amazing what this small physical action can do to ease a patient's anxiety.

2. Simple kindness or a kind word of empathy.

3. Openness and an accepting attitude without any judgment.

4. Asking questions and showing real concern for the person and "not" just the problem.

5. The ability to develop rapport with the patient and playing back "exactly" what a patient has said and then acknowledge that it was heard and understood.

6. Being a good listener and able to acknowledge the person's reason for coming to the dentist.

7. A reassuring manner that may include a caring touch when allowed and appropriate. This includes a gentle touch on the shoulder or taking a patient's hand when noticing their increasing anxiety during treatment.

8. Showing empathy along with compassion and caring.

9. Asking for permission before taking over control and proceeding with any treatment, including an examination.

10. Use stories about yourself and your life to create a distraction from the dental treatment. This may help to develop personal and professional rapport.

> **AUTHOR'S NOTE:** Let me stop here and say that some dentists reading this might shake their heads and not view this list as "tools" needing attention. However, as a former fearful dental patient and after thirty-four years of treating patients with dental anxiety, I have found that the ten items above have helped turn around the dental experiences for a huge number of patients that I have treated. I have also met some colleagues who were very good clinicians but ignored these tools. Then, they wonder why patients did not flock to their practices.

USING PAINLESS TECHNIQUES

I can say that all dentists want to believe that they are painless and that their patients are able to get fully anesthetized and comfortable while in their care.

However, believe it or not, many dentists have had very little experience themselves in the dental chair and are unaware of what it really feels like for their patients. There are also dentists who do not use anesthetic themselves due to a high pain tolerance and a majority of dentists that have never had any dental anxiety. Therefore, they find it difficult to totally understand and empathize with their patients that have high levels of fear.

Those that do accept and understand their patient's fears, invest time and money learning effective techniques. They also offer an assortment of devices to help minimize and hopefully alleviate any pain for their patients.

When a dentist uses painless techniques, they are offering their patients the feeling of safety, confidence and trust that their appointment will go well. Words spread fast and more patients are willing to seek out dental care. Offering and delivering "pain free" dental care not only helps build a dental practice, but also helps our dental profession as a whole.

Each dentist makes his or her own choice. Each knows what works and what "does not" work for them in their own practice. These days there are more than enough options to fit every dentist and every patient's needs.

What might stop a dentist from delivering "pain free" dental care could be a lack of understanding or believing patients when they say they are in pain and feeling the procedure that is being performed.

It is important to remember that there are many types of pain and each of us feel pain differently. I believe, as dentists, we must listen to and believe it when our patients tell us they are feeling pain. Then, it is up to us to address it the best way we can.

Here are fifteen techniques that are available and can be used.

1. The dentist should explain the dental procedure prior to doing it. This allows those patients that may be fearful to mentally and emotionally prepare themselves.

2. Dentists should learn and practice as many painless injection techniques as they can and practice them until skilled.

3. The dentist should inform the patient of all adjunctive aids available for painless injections. Then, choose what works best and what the patient finds most comfortable and useful.

4. The dentist should massage the topical into the area and then shake the patient's lip gently, but firmly, to distract them and their pain centers. This allows the anesthetic to slowly enter into the injection site. This technique has been positively commented on by many of my patients over the years as making their injection painless and bearable.

5. The dentist should use the thinnest needle possible and inject slowly and carefully. According to current dental literature, it should take about sixty seconds to inject one complete carpule. I have found that going slowly and carefully is important. However, for kids and really phobic people, sometimes it is best to take less time.

6. The dentist should re-assure and comfort the patient while injecting and have them "relax their bodies into the chair" while taking slow, deep breaths.

7. The dentist can ask an assistant to hold the patient's hand or be prepared to, if requested.

8. The dentist should inform the patient before beginning any treatment that if he or she needs your attention, they should simply raise their hand.

9. The dentist should stop the treatment when a patient asks.

10. The dentist and the dental assistant should make sure that they place all instruments gently and carefully inside the patient's mouth.

11. The dentist should let the patient know when the procedure is complete and ask the patient how well everything was performed.

12. The dentist should treat the patient as if they were a good friend or a beloved family member.

13. If the patient feels any pain, the dentist should apologize and ask what could have been done to make it better.

14. Some patients need to feel that they are "in control." One technique I have used in my dental practice is a hand held message system. Actually, one of my anxious patients made it for me out of cardboard and construction paper. It had flappable pages with sayings such as: "Stop,""Ouch," "I need a break," "My mouth is tired," "Nice Job Doc" and "I am doing fine."

15. Many patients need to hold onto something for comfort, support and as a tension release. It could be a tissue or paper towel, a blanket or a rubber hand device for release of tension. I had an assortment of these devices in my office over the years. Some were shaped as balls or teeth and some as musical instruments. The guitar shape is my favorite. Many patients prefer to hold onto their cell phones. Just be sure to ask them to keep the ringer turned off during their treatment. I have also had patients use a slinky, play dough or silly putty over the years. My attitude is "whatever comforts my patient and keeps them still and happy allows me to better perform my work more efficiently and safely for all."

MEDITATION AND YOGA

Many patients already know how to meditate and/or use Yoga breathing in order to relax themselves and let go of their anxiety for dental treatment. All the dentist has to do is encourage and allow them to proceed and use what works for them during their appointment. If the dentist has some working knowledge of these techniques, it can be quite helpful as a guide to patients; allowing for an easier, more relaxed dental appointment.

HYPNOSIS AND SELF-HYPNOSIS

It helps if a dentist is open minded and allows these alternative treatment modalities in their operatories. Some patients will do self-hypnosis and all a dentist needs to do is to allow the patient the freedom to do so without any judgment or criticism. It will truly make the procedure go much better for both the patient and the dentist.

If a dentist has working knowledge of how to help a patient achieve a hypnotic state or get into a "zone" of comfort and relaxation, I strongly encourage them to do so. Most of these patients will appreciate a few guided words of reassurance and direction during their treatment.

If a dentist has no such training, has difficulty treating anxious patients or gets stressed just knowing they are scheduled, I urge them to either refer these patients to dentists better skilled to handle them or to become more familiar with this field. It will not only be appreciated by their patients, but it can also benefit the dentist as well.

NLP or NEURO-LINGUISTIC PROGRAMMING

In my private practice I have renamed "Neuro-Linguistic Programming." I call it The Neuro-Linguistic Process or AMC, Anxiety Management Counseling.

According to Lindagail and associates, NLP institute of Oregon, 1995:

"NLP is about Communication. One of the principles of NLP is that we are ALWAYS communicating, and most of our communication is other than words.

NLP is about how language affects us. The very process of converting experience into language requires that we condense, distort, and summarize how we perceive the world. It teaches us to understand how language affects us through implicit and embedded assumptions.

NLP is about modeling excellence. Modeling skills are the heart of NLP. Learning the specific components of how others do something well will provide you with new options.

NLP is how we use our brain. NLP describes in very precise terms, the images, sounds, and feelings that make up our inner world. How do we know what we know? How do we do what we do? NLP is how we code our experience. Sometimes people describe NLP as "software for our brains."

"NLP is the study of internal experience. NLP is a tool to understand how an individual makes sense of the world. NLP studies individual's experiences: how they perceive the world around them and how their brain makes specific distinctions for them. It does not assume that we all do this the same way. NLP is inherently respectful of differences." (Lindagail and associates, NLP institute of Oregon, 1995)

For me, NLP is a process by which the Practitioner or Guide helps someone "go into their own minds," consciously and subconsciously, to discover their current strategies for thinking and functioning. It is a process which can help to determine what is working and what is not. Basically, it's figuring out just how our mind works. It is "a user's guide for our brain."

The Guide offers resources and new tools and strategies to help the person function better. Learning how to use one's brain more effectively can only come about if you first know what you are currently doing and where the blocks, including fears and anxieties, come from.

It is an amazing process. When I was first introduced to it, I was looking for a way to work better with my staff and to become a better communicator and manager.

However, it changed my entire perspective of the world. It not only helped me at work, but also at home with my marriage. I learned incredible techniques and processes to help my fearful and phobic dental patients. I felt like I had hit the jackpot. I not only completed the practitioner's training, but I went on to become a Master Practitioner and then to learn some techniques for being a Health Practitioner.

For a dentist or any individual that tells me that they are struggling at home or at their office with their own stresses and anxieties, I strongly suggest for them to check it out. Even just taking the one day introductory class will open up one's mind to allow you to see the world with a whole new set of eyes, and a new perspective.

Personally, I combine my hypnosis training, (I am a Certified Clinical Hypnotherapist) with my NLP Master training and use it daily in my practice and in my own life.

ANTI-ANXIETY MEDICATIONS

There are many different types of medications used in the treatment of anxiety disorders. Some work better for one person compared to another. I feel that as long as you are under the care of your doctor and dentist, and understand the reason that you are taking it and what to expect, it is definitely a reasonable option when seeking more comfortable dental care.

However, it is very important to remember that although medication can relieve some of the symptoms of anxiety, the medication does not cure the underlying problem. Like all medications, anti-anxiety medications have side effects and safety concerns, including the risk of addiction. So, it is extremely important to discuss taking any medication with your doctor and dentist and to review the pros and cons before deciding.

Here are a couple of approaches that I am familiar with regarding the use of anti-anxiety medications.

1. A patient can take their own anti-anxiety medications like Ativan or Valium or ask their primary care physician to prescribe something for their dental appointment knowing their medical profile.

2. A dentist can prescribe Valium or Lorazepam as a pre-medication if appropriate, knowing the patient's medical history and dental anxiety level. I do suggest that the dentist advise their patient to do a trial test the first time using this method. My patient will take one pill as pre-medication for a simple dental exam appointment or they will do a pre-test and take one pill on a weekend in order to see how that dose affects them. For a minimally anxious patient, one pill may be perfect. However, for a patient with moderate anxiety, two pills or a higher dosage may be required. It is much better to know before the treatment exactly how much medication a patient requires for their restorative appointment.

3. Most of the time I have my moderately anxious patients take one pill the night prior to the dental appointment and then one more pill is taken one hour before they come into the office the following day. Since taking two pills affects the patient's reflexes and state of mind, I always require them to have a companion drive them to and from their appointment.

My motto is: *"Better to be safe than sorry."* I want to protect my patients, my office and myself.

USE OF NITROUS OXIDE (N20)

Nitrous oxide (N20) is also known as "laughing gas" or "nitrous"- This is a safe and effective sedative agent that is a mixture of nitrogen and oxygen and inhaled through a nose mask.

When I was an undergraduate at Tufts University Dental School, we were usually only allowed to use this for pediatric patients (children). However, when I opened up my first dental practice, I found it even more useful and needed for my adult patients, who were either fearful and had been unable to seek dental care or for those who had been traumatized or hurt by a dentist when they were young.

As long as a dentist is well trained, aware of all the risks and precautions for themselves, their staff and their patients and have a fail-safe system (which the newer systems are), it can be an excellent tool to have in your "Dental Anti-Anxiety" toolkit. There is also the side benefit of it being a terrific practice builder.

WHY DENTISTS SHOULD USE N20 WITH CAUTION

I always caution other dentists to ask their patients if they have ever had nitrous oxide and what was their prior experience. If it was a positive one, try to replicate what worked. If it was not so pleasant, find out what happened and make their next time a good experience or choose another technique.

Whatever you do, never push a patient into using it. If a patient offers real resistance, not just their fear of the unknown, listen to them and "trust" their decision. You must respect it and find another option. Some patients have had a bad experience of getting nauseous or dizzy and vomiting and will not want to try it ever again, I have found that, in many cases, it was due to a "too high" a percentage of the nitrous used in the N20 mixture.

Also, after the procedure is completed, check your patient very carefully before you release them from the office. Some patients may still feel a little woozy or "off center" and should be allowed to sit a while longer until their minds are fully clear and feel safe enough to drive home.

MY PERSONAL EXPERIENCE WITH N20

Recently, I used N20 for a patient who was trying it for the first time for an extraction (removing a tooth). I removed the nose mask after giving him fifteen minutes of oxygen and had him sit for fifteen minutes more before bringing him to the front reception area. The procedure had gone beautifully and he told me it was a good experience for him and helped him immensely. We walked him out to the reception area and he asked to sit down a little longer, indicating that he needed to clear his head before he drove home. After another 20 minutes, he told our receptionist that he felt much better and was going home. When he came in the following week for his post-operative appointment, he shared with me that he was a "lightweight." He said he left our office feeling totally like himself and got into his car to drive home. When he came to a rotary (traffic circle) he couldn't quite figure out what lane he was supposed to be in and almost had an accident. It totally surprised him and made him aware that in the future he would ask a companion to drive him to any appointment where he was using nitrous oxide.

I have found that most of my patients have had "no" post sedative affects when only nitrous oxide has been used. However, this situation reminds me that each patient is unique and medications, including "laughing gas" can affect them differently.

In this regard, a dentist and his or her staff must watch their patients carefully and keep them safe at all times.

For those dentists not currently using nitrous oxide, please do not let these possible side effects stop you from learning this incredibly safe and easy adjunct for patients with dental anxiety.
I discovered that years ago, many dentists felt that "more is better" when using nitrous and used 50% and even higher as the norm for all their patients. Although this can be highly effective for some patients, especially children, I have found that it is much too high for most adults and can make them sick and nauseous. Children seem to do well with 50% as a rule, but even then it is safer to stay at the 30-40% range until you are sure.

Then, there are those patients that need a minimal dose and can do well between 10-30%, while others may need 60% or higher. Some even say they cannot feel any difference in their mental state with the 70% range.

The best technique that I have found to use with a new patient is to explain the process before I place the mask on them. I ask questions and give clear, concise directions and help them get acclimated. Then, I add in some suggestions for meditating or visioning using hypnotic language as I turn on the nitrous oxide system and watch them closely. I calibrate my patient (noticing any and all changes), watching closely how their eyes, face, breathing and entire body is reacting and slowly raise the percentage to 40% or higher if needed. I continue to communicate with them along the way and remind them that they are in control. If they want more or less or want the mask removed completely, all they have to do is signal me with their left hand.

I give each patient 5-10 minutes of pure oxygen to start with to get them used to breathing the way I want them to and to prepare their bodies. I also end their appointment with 5-15 minutes of pure oxygen, depending on how long they were on the nitrous in order to clean out their system, get them alert and able to leave my office safely.

THREE BAD REACTIONS

I have had only three bad reactions to using nitrous in my thirty-four years of practice (Hopefully, this will be all, but as Murphy's Law predicts, there is most likely another one in my future).

1. Just after graduating from dental school, I used nitrous at 30-40% for a new patient, but did not ask enough questions about the man's personal history. I also had no experience yet in NLP or Hypnosis. My patient was on the nitrous for about 10 minutes, when all of a sudden he tore off the mask and ran into the corner of my operatory. I could see that his body was shaking and he was completely hunched over and hugging himself into a ball as he rocked back and forth.

   You can imagine how shocked I was. I was so new to it all that I didn't know what I had done, if anything. Being a trained professional, I stayed as calm as I could, went immediately over to him, spoke softly and asked if he was okay. I put out my hand in case he wanted comfort and grounding, but did not touch him. He opened up his eyes and looked at me and said, "I'm okay. Give me some time. I'm really okay, now."

   I waited with him on the floor and within five minutes he sat up. He then told me that he was a "Vietnam War Veteran" and the nitrous had allowed him to remember a blocked out memory that usually only came out at night when he was sleeping. He had been diagnosed with PTSD,

(Post Traumatic Stress Disorder), but hadn't thought it was important to mention it on his health history.
Well, that was a lesson for both of us.

2. The second incident was years later when a patient told me she wasn't feeling anything at 30%. It appeared that her prior use of anti-anxiety medications may have blocked her sensitivity to nitrous. She had warned me of her high tolerance to most medications. I decided to raise her nitrous level to 40% and seeing little change, I raised it to 45%. All of a sudden she began to breathe fast and furious and became agitated in the chair. She told me she was becoming more anxious and needed it turned off. I immediately turned off the flow of the nitrogen completely and raised the oxygen level and helped her by guiding her to take slow, deep breaths and to allow her anxiety to pass as the oxygen coursed through her body. I took off the mask and she told me that she was fine and requested that I complete the procedure, since she was already anesthetized. I calibrated that she truly was okay and it was safe to continue.

3. The third time I had a bad reaction was while treating a Non-IV Oral Conscious Sedation patient (OCS). [See pages 88-90 for more information on this process]. My patient was getting relaxed and in a semi sleeping state. I decided to leave the nitrous on at 40% and proceed with her treatment. About half way into my procedure she awoke and told me she was going to be sick. My assistant quickly got the emesis basin, the patient vomited while I helped her get calm and back to a comfortable state. I had already turned off the nitrogen and raised the oxygen to

100%. After a few minutes she said she was fine and I calibrated that indeed she was. She asked me to continue with her treatment, which I did using only oxygen and she had no additional problems. When I saw her at her post-operative appointment, she was fine and had no memory of the nausea and vomiting. As a matter of fact, she thanked me and told me it had been a good experience and she would do it again when she needed more dental work. From that time on, I began to lower my nitrous to between 10-30% during the OCS process, depending on how sedated my patient was, what procedures I was doing, and what percentage would be optimum for each person's comfort. Some OCS patients need only the pure oxygen once they are relaxed and comfortable.

It is important to mention that this was the first and only time that one of my sedation patients actually vomited. So, my fellow dentists and anxious patients reading this please do not let this scare you off from considering it.

Since that time, I have added another medication called Hydroxyzine to my OCS protocol. Hydroxyzine helps decrease the possibility of nausea and intensifies the sedation experience. I use this for a majority of my patients when I feel it will be beneficial.

> **AUTHOR'S NOTE:** For anyone considering having Non-IV Oral Conscious Sedation for their dental care, it is a very common experience to have amnesia and no memory of the actual dental treatment. Actually, that is one of the most favorable side effects of the process.

NITROUS OXIDE WITH VALIUM

I consider this combination a light to moderate sedation technique.

Many patients find that using either of these alone do not give them the comfort and release from anxiety required and therefore need the combination of the two to reach the desired effect. I have found that the pre-medication with Valium starts to take effect about the time the nitrous level is perfect for the patient. The nitrous also changes the patient's internal experience in a way that allows the Valium to be more effective. It is the dentist's responsibility to know their patients well enough and to be able to calibrate just how much Valium to give each patient and what percentage of nitrous oxide to use.

USE OF ALCOHOL

When I first began practicing, the idea of any patient having alcohol before their dental appointment was totally unacceptable to me. However, as time has passed, I have become much more experienced and open-minded. I have had a handful of patients tell me that taking a drink before their dental appointment helps them with their dental anxiety. As long as the patient and I have developed a treatment plan, are in agreement as to what each appointment will entail and they inform me as to exactly what they drank before I begin any treatment, then I am comfortable treating them. I also ask them to have a companion drive them to and from their appointments.

Let me clearly say that this mutual consent is quite different from a patient coming in drunk or high. I handle those issues very differently.

USE OF MUSIC AND HEADPHONES

I have seen many patients settle down and relax in a dental chair with only the use of an I-Phone, MP3 player or CD player with music. It seems that when the audio channel in a patients mind is filled with music or a tape or an audio book, it blocks the conscious mind from thinking anxious thoughts and allows them to relax and release their inner anxiety. It may start off as a distraction, but it turns into an enjoyable experience. I actually encourage many of my patients to use the headphones and to listen to whatever comforts them in order to block out the sounds of the drill. This is a novel idea to many people, but when they try it they tell me it is effective and works well.

NON-IV ORAL CONSCIOUS SEDATION (OCS)

This type of moderate sedation allows a patient to be in a semi-sleeping, semi-conscious state to have their dental treatment done and have little or no memory the day after. This one technique has made a huge difference in my second practice. It has made dental care available to many more patients who would have either not sought care or would have only gone to an oral surgeon for extractions, whereby potentially leaving them a "dental cripple."

This technique was not readily available to me or my patients in my first dental practice in Boise, Idaho. When a patient came to see me who was so filled with anxiety and told me they had to be "knocked out completely" in order to get any treatment, the only option available to me was to refer them to an oral surgeon or to seek dental care in a hospital setting. Since there were no dental schools in Idaho, it left very little choice for my phobic patients.

When I moved to Massachusetts and learned about a new organization called DOCS Education (Dental Organization for Conscious Sedation), I immediately checked them out and signed up for the first course offered. They are an amazing group of physicians and dentists offering numerous continuing education courses in Conscious Sedation for adults and children. I have since attended many of their courses and many others elsewhere in order to keep current and offer the best care possible.

Once I became fully licensed to practice this type of sedation in my office, I began using the following protocol.

1. We schedule a sedation consult with the patient a few days to one week prior to the treatment appointment.

2. For their first sedation experience, we also like to have the patient's companion present at the consult if at all possible.

3. We fully review their health history again, review the procedures being done, the sedation process and get all the necessary consents signed.

4. We make sure the patient and their companion fully understand and consent to all the requirements and procedures before, during and after treatment.

5. My patient will then take either Valium or Lorazepam the night prior to the sedation appointment. Then, in the morning they take one tablet of 0.25 mg Triazolam (Halcion) one hour prior to their dental appointment and are driven by their companion to my office. They are not allowed to drive once they have taken their Triazolam (sleeping pill). In my office we are extremely protective and cautious with our patients undergoing sedation.

6. On the treatment day, we review the instructions with the patient and companion, settle our patient into a chair with specially designed miracle foam padding for their comfort, and I determine how much more medication my patient requires in order to achieve the optimum state needed for their treatment.

7. Usually, I give the patient an additional 0.25 mg or 0.50 mg Triazolam under their tongue and add in 25 mg Hydroxyzine (this will minimize any possible nausea and enhance the sedation experience) and let them rest with the lights out for about 20-30 minutes. I also encourage the use of and provide them a compact disc player and headphones prior to starting the nitrous oxide. When the treatment is completed, I turn down the nitrogen and use only the oxygen for 10-15 minutes to flush out their system and prepare them for leaving the office.

8. Then, I remove the mask, sit the patient upright and give them some juice and liquid nutrition to allow them to come back from their sleeping state. I tell my patient how well they did, review the treatment done and the post-operative instructions with their companion and wheel our patient in a wheelchair to their waiting vehicle.

Let me reiterate that not only does this protocol facilitate a pleasant visit for the patient, but it has a wonderful amnesic effect giving the patient little or no memory of the appointment the following day. I also like the fact that we can safely reverse the sedation process by a reversal agent if an emergency develops. This technique has helped many, many patients not only save their teeth and get incredible amounts of dentistry accomplished, but it has also increased many a person's self-esteem while improving their lives.

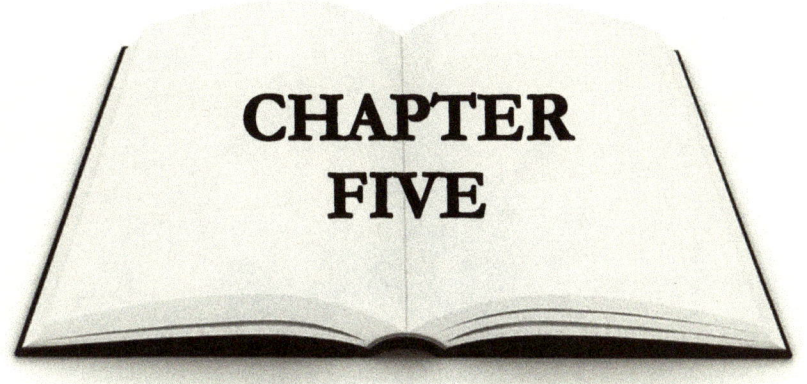

HYPNOSIS AND ACUPUNCTURE

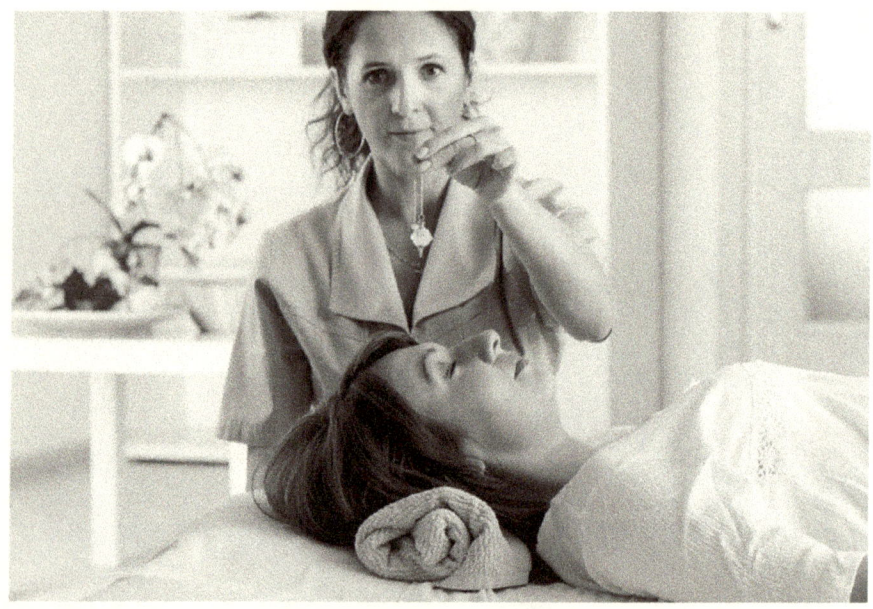

"Hypnosis has been described as an altered awareness, a state of relaxation or a detachment from the current environment."

HYPNOSIS

The Journal of The Massachusetts Dental Society had an excellent description of hypnosis in their winter 1999 magazine on page nine. In an article titled "Using Mind-Body Techniques in Dentistry," by Eleanor F. Counselman, ED.D, ABPP, She wrote:

"Hypnosis is probably the best known (and possibly most feared) mind-body technique. Hypnosis is an intensified state of concentration. Individuals in this state, or trance, are more attentive and receptive to suggestions. Hypnosis does not place the hypnotized individual under the power of the hypnotist. In fact, all hypnosis is really self-hypnosis. (Spiegel H, Spiegel D. Trance and Treatment. Washington, DC: American Psychiatric Press; 1978)

The hypnotist simply serves as a facilitator to help the subject learn how to enter and deepen the trance-state and how to effectively work with affirmations, imagery, and post-hypnotic suggestions. It is not possible for hypnotized individuals to do some-thing against their will.

Approximately four out of five patients can be hypnotized to some degree."

HYPNOSIS IN DENTISTRY

Hypnosis has been described as "an altered awareness", "a state of relaxation" or a "detachment from the current environment." In my dental setting, I call it "getting into a zone where one feels safe, protected, comfortable and calm."

In a 1978 article titled "Spiegel D. Trance and Treatment" in American Psychiatric Press, Dr. Spiegel states, "Hypnosis is actually a state of intense concentration with a reduction in peripheral awareness." He also says that, "like a telephoto rather than a wide angle lens. You stay completely in control. Doctors call the creation of that dual reality *Disassociation,* and although you may achieve it spontaneously, hypnosis teaches you to do it at will."

In a 1988 article in Glamour Magazine (pages 72-78), Ginny Graves says "If you ever zone out while driving or been so caught up in a movie that you felt disoriented leaving the theater, you've experienced a trance state." In the same magazine, Dr. Moshe Torem states, "In hypnosis you're so absorbed in whatever you're thinking about that you aren't aware of your physical surroundings" and Dr. Spiegel says that he believes: "The part of the brain involved in focusing your attention may simply give priority to something else." He states, "Doctors call the creation of that dual reality "Disassociation", and although you may achieve it spontaneously, hypnosis teaches you to do it at will."

In the same issue of Glamour Magazine, I found this quote, "It has been said that eighty percent of people are hypnotizable to some extent."

AUTHOR'S NOTE: A suggestion I was given a while ago for "needle phobic" dental patients can be used when being giving an injection. The patient focuses on a "feeling of icy cold". This directs your conscious mind to perceive and feel the needle differently and less "scary."

In the Academy of General Dentistry Impact Magazine (July 1994, page 11), it was written that: "During hypnosis, patients display physical and mental relaxation, full regular breathing and a decrease in tension and anxiety." Some patients cannot be hypnotized. If a patient is resistant to hypnosis, the technique will not work." The patient needs to be highly motivated and there needs to be a level of cooperation by the patient."

On page 9 of the same magazine it states "Dentists who provide hypnosis for their patients often resort to the techniques for themselves to reduce their own stress and to avoid transmitting stress."

"The nature of the dental treatment brings us (dentists), into close proximity with the patient, and we're bombarded with powerful negative emotional feelings of fear and hostility," says Dr. Rausch.

"Dentists are generally a stressed out group. We deal with patients who are very often hostile and fearful. I use self-hypnosis at chairside to become really focused on what I'm doing. I find it relaxing" says Margaret McCaulley, DDS. (Academy of General Dentistry Impact, July 1994, page 9)

Here are some interesting references about using Hypnosis as an adjunct in medical treatment:

- Harold Golan, DMD says that a few of his patients came to him for hypnosis as a last resort. "Through hypnosis, his patients were able to avoid surgery." (Academy of General Dentistry Impact, July 1994, page 9)

- L. Henry Clark, DMD says he "regularly uses hypnosis with patients who are allergic to anesthesia, are dental phobics or who want to avoid anesthesia." (Academy of General Dentistry Impact, July 1994, page 9)

- In the April 1988 edition of Glamour Magazine, (pages 72-78) there was an article called *Can Hypnosis Make You Healthier?* The article states, "Doctors now say hypnotic suggestion can be as effective as drugs and surgery for some problems and there are no side effects."

ACUPUNCTURE

Here is the best definition of acupuncture I could find.

"Acupuncture is a treatment method that involves the painless insertion of very fine needles into highly specific points in the skin. It is valuable in relieving toothaches, because it is natural and does not involve drugs", says Frank Yurasek, MA, Acupuncturist. "Used synergistically with dentistry, it can be used for pain relief in the oral cavity, stress management and healing promotion." (Academy of General Dentistry Impact, October 1993, page 14)

AUTHOR'S NOTE: Although I have never employed this technique myself, I have had some patients tell me that they have used Acupuncture for their prior dental treatment and found it extremely effective.

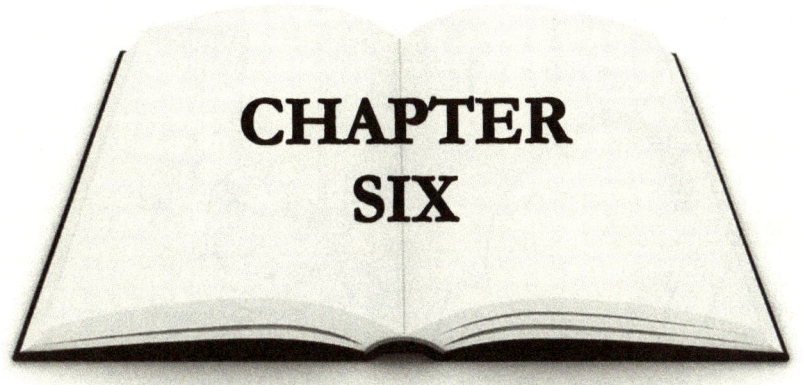

CHAPTER SIX

BARRIERS TO GETTING DENTAL CARE FOR FEARFUL PATIENTS

Why are the Statistics of People Afraid to go to the Dentist Still So High?

HAVE NO FEAR OF THE DENTAL CHAIR!

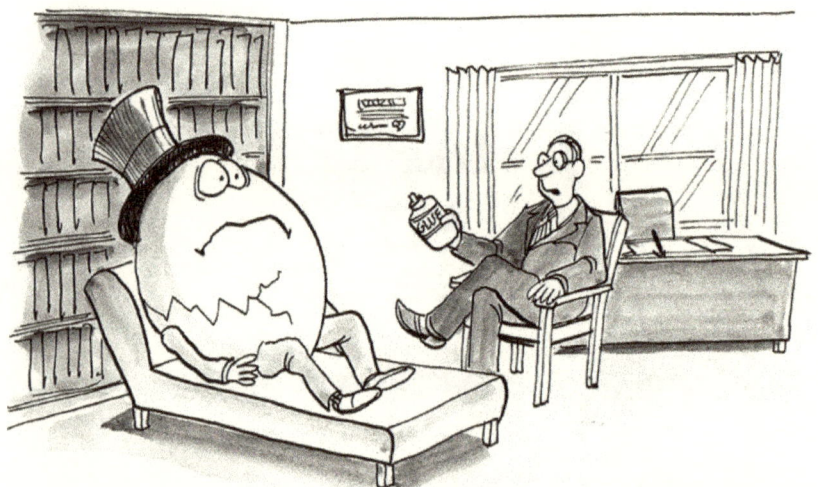

"Visualize yourself not falling off the wall."

BARRIERS TO GETTING DENTAL CARE

I have found that the more relaxed my patient is the easier and faster I can perform their treatment. When a patient is relaxed the anesthetic works better and the dentist can work more efficiently focusing on the dental treatment instead of on managing the patient's anxiety. A relaxed patient is a happy patient.

Having any type of anxiety about dentistry will make the decision to schedule an appointment much more difficult. Many of my fearful patients have told me they always wait until their pain is worse than the pain they anticipate at the dental office. Some tell me, *"I just couldn't stand the pain anymore, so here I am."* When they come in to see me, I can see the dread in their eyes or the tears dripping from their lashes or feel their intense fear coming off of their bodies.

Over the years I have identified some of the most common barriers that stop anxious patients from getting the dental care they need. Here is a list of some of these barriers.

THE MOST COMMON BARRIERS

- ✓ Stigma from society in general. These include the following:
  - "You need a nice smile to be successful"
  - An individual's first impression and therefore their judgment of others comes from the condition of one's teeth
- ✓ Society, in general, expects everyone to have a clean, healthy mouth.

- ✓ There is still some fear of dentists proliferated on TV and various advertising venues.
- ✓ Just having fear in and of itself, no matter what kind.
- ✓ Control issues and lack of it.
- ✓ Movies showing negative images of pain at the hands of dentists.
- ✓ Safety issues.
- ✓ Boundary issues.
- ✓ Difficulty saying what they want and standing up for themselves with authority figures.
- ✓ Pain worries and Cost concerns.
- ✓ Education and personal dental IQ status.
- ✓ Learned fear from family or friends.
- ✓ Learned beliefs (including "old wife's tales" of dentists and pain).
- ✓ Learned dental neglect.
- ✓ Past dentistry is different from modern dentistry, but bad rap still exists.
- ✓ The statistics are relatively high of the numbers of people afraid and unable to go to the dentist.
- ✓ Feeling "forced" to go to the dentist or being "shamed" into going.
- ✓ Difficulty finding a dentist adequately prepared and able to handle intensely fearful patients.

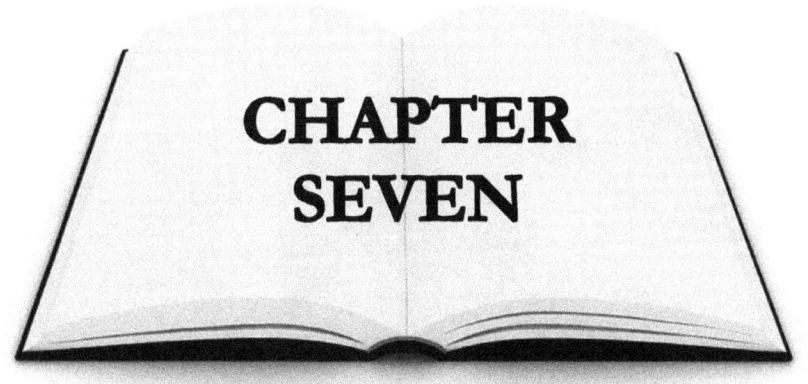

CHAPTER SEVEN

SPECIFIC NEEDS OF A FEARFUL DENTAL PATIENT

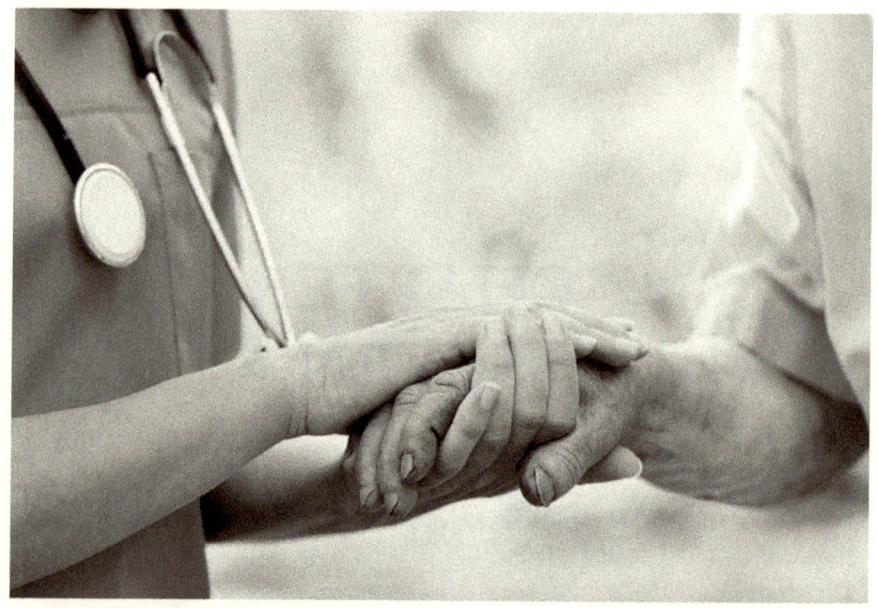

"Being able to relax by blocking out the drill noises, by meditating, wearing headphones, using the nitrous oxide or by whatever means works for them."

SPECIFIC NEEDS OF A FEARFUL DENTAL PATIENT

It is the dentist's responsibility to not only offer excellent dental care, but to also provide their patient with a safe, comfortable environment.

If the dentist understands what their patient's emotional status is and can provide what that individual patient needs, a lot can get accomplished.

Some Specific needs are as follows:

- ❖ Strong rapport with dentist and staff.
- ❖ Education and understanding of dental treatment provided.
- ❖ To be able to feel they can trust the dentist and staff.
- ❖ Feeling cared about as an individual.
- ❖ Feeling understood as to what their concerns, needs and desires are.
- ❖ To be able to feel comfortable with the dentist and staff and not feel like they are being seen "through a microscope."
- ❖ The ability to be able to make their needs known and have them respected.
- ❖ The ability to have or be given some control over their treatment plan, the treatment decisions and the actual treatment while in progress (i.e. taking a break when needed, asking a question mid-treatment).

- ❖ Being able to relax by blocking out the drill noises, by meditating, wearing headphones, using the nitrous oxide or by whatever means works for them.
- ❖ Being able to let someone into their personal and intimate space.
- ❖ The need to feel accepted as belonging, regardless of their emotional state.
- ❖ The need to feel as comfortable as is reasonable in a medical setting.
- ❖ The need to experience no pain or as little discomfort as possible. It is very important to be fully honest and up front with the patient as to what he or she should expect.
- ❖ The need for the dentist to really listen to them and their desires, do the treatment requested and stop immediately when asked. It is very important to be fully honest and up front with patients as to what they should reasonably expect.

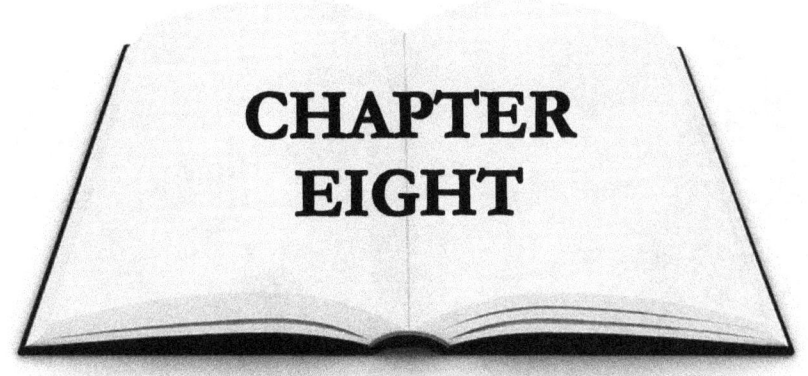

CHAPTER EIGHT

WHAT CAN LEAD TO OR TURN INTO DENTAL ANXIETY?

Fear Responses and Triggers

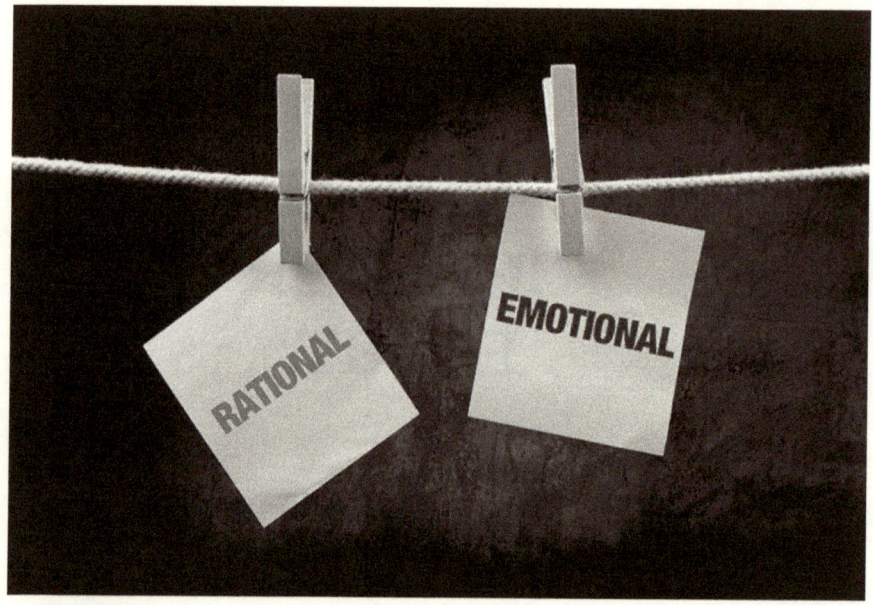

According to the Journal of the American Dental Association, *"Dental patients with a history of traumatic experiences are more likely to engage in negative health habits and to display fear of routine dental care."*

FEAR RESPONSES

The Journal of the American Dental Association or JADA is one of the best sources that I have found that sheds some new insight into what leads to increasing anxiety in dental patients. In this chapter I will just share with you a recent discussion from a JADA 145 article.

In JADA, the following was reported:

"Dental patients with a history of traumatic experiences are more likely to engage in negative health habits and to display fear of routine dental care.

Examples of traumatic life events may include child abuse or neglect, domestic violence, sexual assault, elder abuse and exposure to combat.

Adult victims may respond with fear, anxiety, helplessness or horror and children may respond with feelings of disorganization or agitation.

All of these traumas involve violation of a person's bodily integrity and may influence his or her attitudes toward medical and dental care.

Psychological factors such as anxiety and depression contribute to rescheduled, missed or cancelled appointments. In addition to emotional distress, patients often experience psychological reactions when trauma memories are triggered.

Common fears reported by victims include the following:

(1) Having to lie down for treatment;

(2) Having objects put into their mouth;

(3) The dentist's hand over their mouth or nose;

(4) Not being able to breathe or swallow; and

(5) Worrying that the dentist may get angry.

Thus, dental care related phobia cannot be seen simply as fear of pain and needles."

Now, according to an article from Time Magazine titled, *"What Scares You?,"* (April 2, 2001, pages 50-62), I found the following:

> *"Experts say a True Phobic reaction is a whole different category of terror, a central nervous system wildfire that's impossible to mistake. In the face of the thing that triggers fear, phobics experience sweating, racing heart, difficulty breathing and even a fear of imminent death- all accompanied by an overwhelming need to flee. In addition, much of their time that they are away from the feared object or situation is spent dreading the next encounter and developing elaborate strategies intended to avoid it.*
>
> *It has been written that as many as 40% of all people suffering from a specific phobia have at least one phobic parent.*
>
> *A childhood trauma may be more than enough to seize the brain's attention and serve as a respiratory for incipient fears.*
>
> *What turns up the wattage of a phobia the most is the strategy the phobic rely on to ease their discomfort: Avoidance. The harder a phobic works to avoid the things they fear, the more the brain grows convinced that the threat is real. The things you do to reduce anxiety just makes it worse.*
>
> *Like all other emotional disorders, phobias cause a double dip of psychic pain: from the condition and from the shame of having the problem in the first place.*
>
> *Phobias can beat the stuffing out of the sufferers because the feelings they generate seem so real and the dangers they warn of so great, Most of the time, however, the dangers are more neurochemical lies- and the lies have to be exposed.*

But what you really need to do is face down the fear. When you spend your time in cautionary crouch, the greatest relief of all may come from simply standing up."

FEAR RESPONSES VARY

The Journal of the American Dental Association [JADA (145 (3) page 238] suggests that, interestingly enough, there are some things that can either help or create anxiety in a patient. The Journal states the following:

"A mouth prop can help a patient stay open, but can also cause a patient to feel anxious and powerless when they can't close their mouth;

Saliva ejectors may make a patient feel out of breath and can trigger feelings of panic; and

Oral cancer screenings can reassure some patients, while abuse victims might experience it as forceful and invasive."

Here are a couple of other facts from General Dentistry, May-June 1994, page 237:

"An allergic reaction of a skin rash could be a response to extreme embarrassment.

Also, experiments have shown that people who get urticarial, skin rashes, are a more anxious and depressed group; showing once again that psychological factors can produce severe symptoms."

TRIGGERS

Triggers can set off many emotions, including anxiety and fear. A trigger is usually an external event that causes us to react, respond or feel a certain way without any conscious awareness.

Think to yourself, *"What is the unconscious thought, idea, feeling or internal process that gets me to react the way I do?"* You might think of it as *"What pushes my buttons?"*

There are positive triggers that remind us of good events and moments in our lives and there are the kind of triggers that evoke negative feelings and memories. We may not be aware or conscious of exactly what these are but our minds are like powerful computers. They link sights, sounds, smells, touch and taste with feelings, thoughts and memories. They link our senses-- and we remember.

A person may not understand why they feel afraid of the dentist or have anxiety about dental appointments, but it could be triggering a memory recorded deep within them. This is where NLP, (Neuro-Linguistic Programming), hypnosis or speaking with a therapist or counselor can be extremely helpful in uncovering and eventually releasing those triggers and hidden memories.

CHAPTER NINE

WHAT CAN ANXIOUS PATIENTS DO TO PREPARE FOR A DENTAL APPOINTMENT?

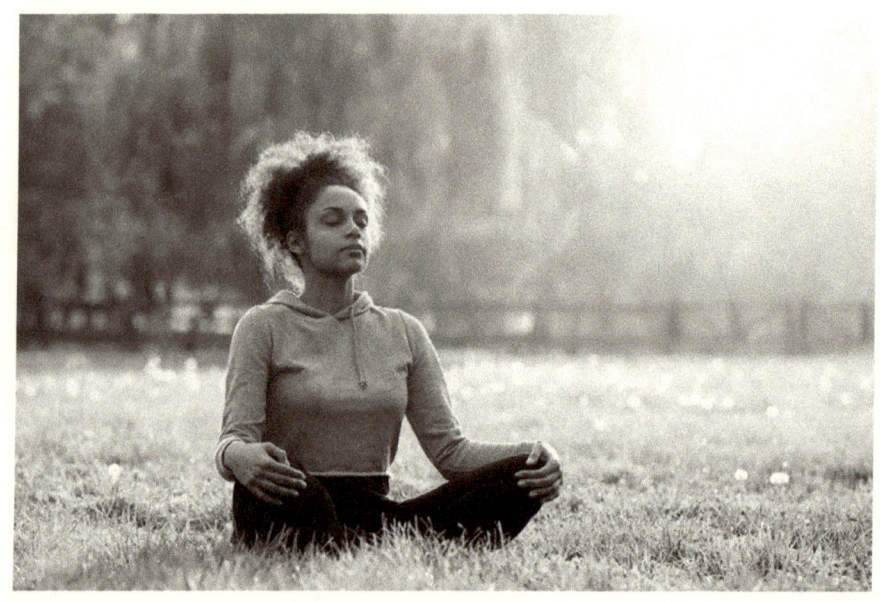

"Practice meditation or visioning or yoga breathing before you go, to mentally prepare yourself for the appointment."

WHY IT IS IMPORTANT TO BE PREPARED?

As with any undertaking, the better prepared you are, the better the outcome. Many years ago I was told: "If you fail to plan, then plan to fail!" (Benjamin Franklin). The same is true for dental appointments, especially if anxiety is involved.

For most patients the planning involves scheduling an appointment, arranging time off from work, getting day care for children, arranging transportation, packing an insurance card and credit card or checkbook. These are almost second nature for going to a medical, dental or healthcare appointment. However, for an anxious patient, who could be obsessing or panicking days prior to their appointment, there is much more that can and should be done to give them peace of mind and help prepare them for a positive dental experience.

WHAT YOU CAN DO TO BE PREPARED

- Check out your dentist carefully. This can be done by a phone contact, internet search, asking trusted friends and family, asking medical professionals and getting a referral from your own doctors.
- Schedule an appointment for only a consultation, if the idea of having an actual dental appointment is too stressful. Then, decide if this is a dentist you can work with, communicate with and ultimately trust to not only do good dentistry but to treat you well and not hurt you.
- Schedule a cleaning appointment to check out the office environment and the hygienist's "touch." This will allow you to gain a sense of the dentist's choice of staff and

office setting and to determine if you feel comfortable there.

➢ Put together your list of concerns and questions to ask about the type of care you expect and your personal needs and desires.

➢ Practice meditation, visioning or yoga breathing before you go, to mentally prepare yourself for the appointment.

➢ Consider taking a self-hypnosis class or learn whatever relaxation techniques you think will help reduce your anxiety.

➢ Take your usual anxiety medication prior to your dental appointment or call your General Practitioner for pre-medication (Be sure you tell the dentist what medication you have taken).

➢ Bring an I-Phone, MP3 or CD player with a set of headphones to listen to and help block out the dental sounds. This will allow you to relax into yourself during the appointment.

➢ Bring your blanket or any other comfort to hold onto during the appointment.

➢ Plan to dress for "your" personal comfort.

➢ Go to a therapist or counselor before your dental appointment for help in preparing for and learning ways to get through your time at the dental office.

➢ Practice imagining in your mind how comfortable and easy your appointment will be (visioning). This may help you feel ready and comfortable enough to schedule an actual appointment. Then, go in expecting the appointment will go well.

- ➤ Share honestly with an understanding friend about your worries and anxieties and ask them to accompany you as your "security blanket."
- ➤ For those that believe in a "Higher Power", use your faith and the power of prayer to remind you that you are not doing it all alone. Before the appointment and also at the dental office, you can ask for help from your spiritual source to watch over you and help empower your inner reserve of strength.
- ➤ According to a dental article published by the AGD Impact Magazine, (February 2015), you should avoid caffeine and sugar before your dental appointment because they could increase your anxiety.

HAVE NO FEAR OF THE DENTAL CHAIR!

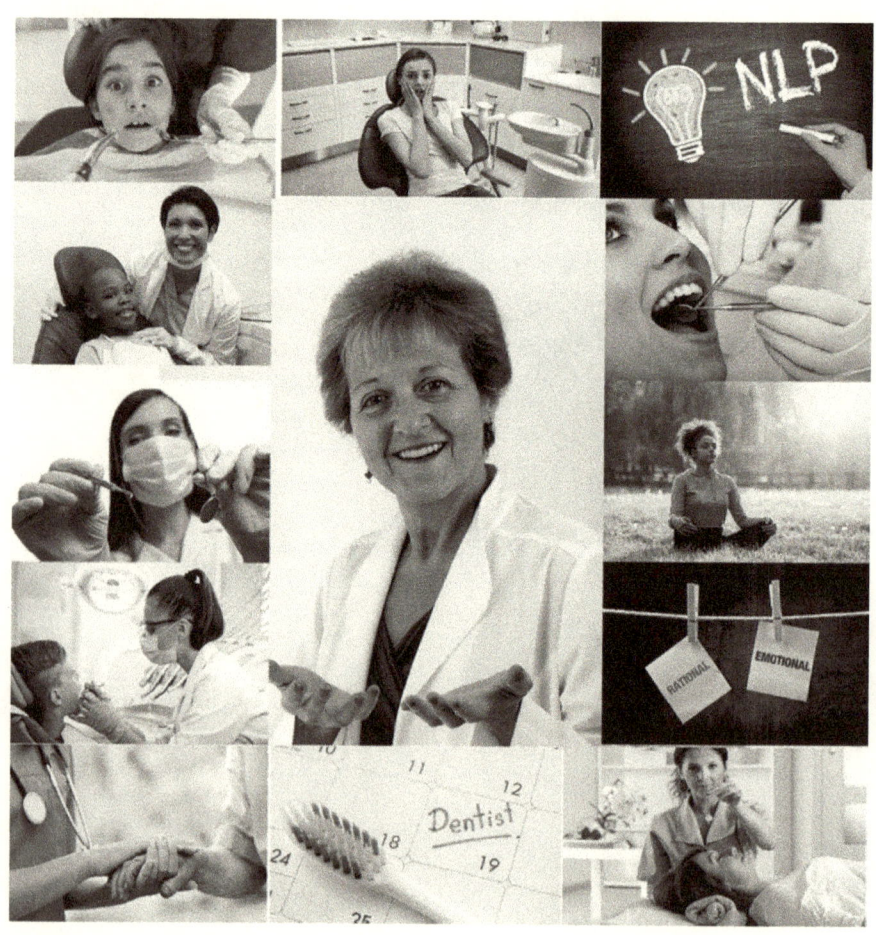

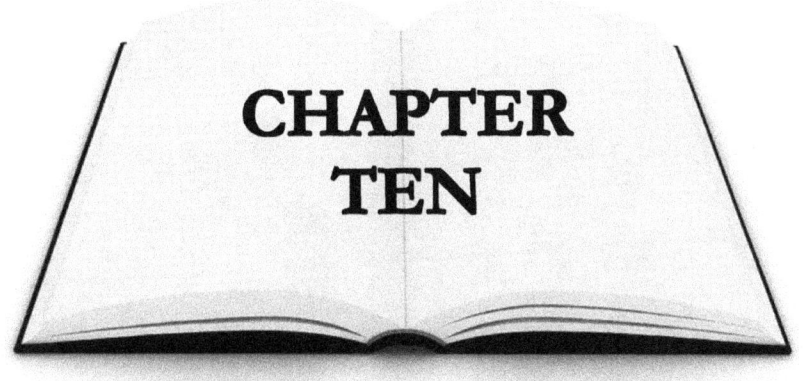

CHAPTER TEN

WHAT CAN ANXIOUS PATIENTS DO TO HELP THEMSELVES AT THE DENTAL APPOINTMENT?

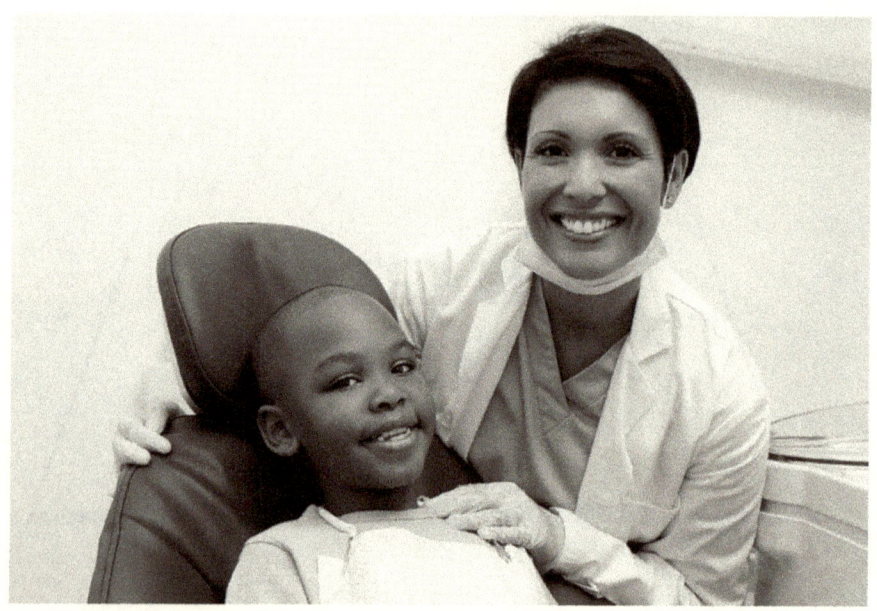

"You as a dental patient or parent must take personal responsibility and learn more about yourself or your child and what is needed. Consider what you have tried and what worked and what didn't work and share it with the dental staff."

HOW TO HELP YOURSELF DURING THE DENTAL APPOINTMENT

Once you as a patient have scheduled an appointment and "gotten all your ducks in a row" via the planning process, then, it helps to have definitive tools to use once you are in the dental office and ready to be treated.

Here are some things you can do to help yourself during the dental appointment:

- ✓ Let the receptionist, dental assistant and the dentist know that you are anxious and at what level, (scale of 1-10).
- ✓ Ask about the procedure being done and request as much information as you need (i.e. How long will the drilling take and What time will you be done?).
- ✓ Tell the dentist and staff what you need.
    - Do you need to not see any of the dental instruments, including the needle?
    - Do you need to know or not know what is going on during the treatment?
    - Do you have any issues with specific anesthetics or having your mouth open too long?
    - Do you need your hand held during the anesthetic process?
    - Do you need or want nitrous oxide or a mouth prop for treatment?
- ✓ Ask for topical anesthetic before any injection, in case the dentist does not offer it or use it routinely.
- ✓ Be proactive and listen to music or an audio book at the appointment.

- ✓ Ask for a blanket or a pillow for comfort or bring your own.
- ✓ Keep your eyes closed during the dental treatment and imagine something that comforts you or relaxes you.
- ✓ Meditate or do Yoga breathing (remember to focus on your breathing and do not hold your breath. If you do your oxygen levels will decrease, which increases anxiety).
- ✓ Use self-hypnosis.
- ✓ Tell the dentist if you need additional anesthetic or a time out. You have a voice. You should work out a sign with the dentist ahead of time-before the treatment has begun.
- ✓ Try to remember: "It will all be over soon."
- ✓ Remember, you are actually in control and can ask the dentist to stop at any time. You are not a victim or powerless.
- ✓ Remember you are now an adult and no longer a helpless, scared child (for those with trauma from childhood).

AUTHOR'S NOTE: There are many ways for a patient to communicate with a dentist. During my 34 years of treating patients, I have used numerous techniques and tools to help my patient in the chair. Some have worked better than others. Some patients like one technique better than another or some not at all. You as a dental patient "must" take personal responsibility and learn more about yourself and what you need. Consider what you have tried and what worked and what didn't work and share it with the dental staff.

HOW A PATIENT CAN "STAY IN CONTROL"

According to Romeo Vitelli, Ph.D. (Psychology Today, Media Spotlight, Staying in Control, posted October 21, 2013), *"The confidence we have in our ability to control our own lives plays an important role in maintaining a healthy lifestyle."*

Dr. Vitelli defined perceived control as "The belief that one has the ability to make a difference in the course or the consequences of some event or experience, often helpful in dealing with stressors." He adds that "perceived control may also influence how we regulate emotions and handle stress that can help us cope more effectively."

I have found that when I feel like I have some control in a given situation, I not only feel more courageous and able to take a risk, but I also feel more confident in my ability to stand up for myself and ask for what I need.

This has also been the case for those patients I have guided and counseled with over the years. I have witnessed many patients taking control during their dental appointments. This control allowed them to have a much better dental experience and procedure outcome.

Here are some ways to "stay in control" during the dental appointment:

- Be honest and use your voice to tell the dentist and staff what you need in order to feel safe and less afraid.
- Develop trust with your dentist and staff and communicate.
- Call the office before your appointment to be reassured and remind them again when you get to the appointment of your dental anxiety.

- Only do as much treatment at your appointment as you can handle.
- Use your agreed upon "hand signal" if you have something to say or need a break.
- Ask a trusted companion to bring you and take you home.
- Remember that you are not a victim! You are an adult and not a helpless child.

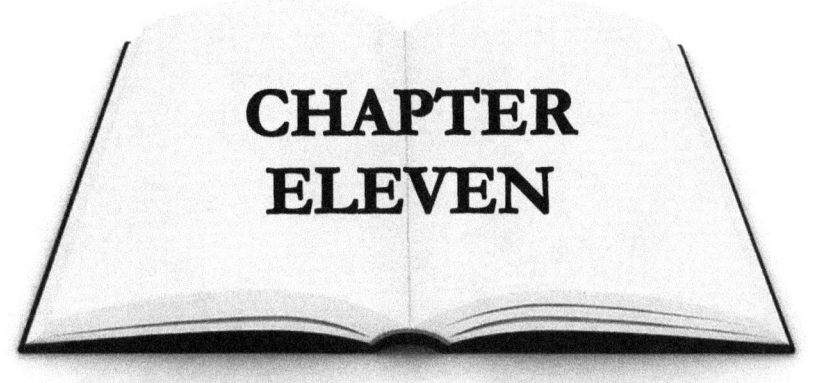

CHAPTER ELEVEN

GAGGING

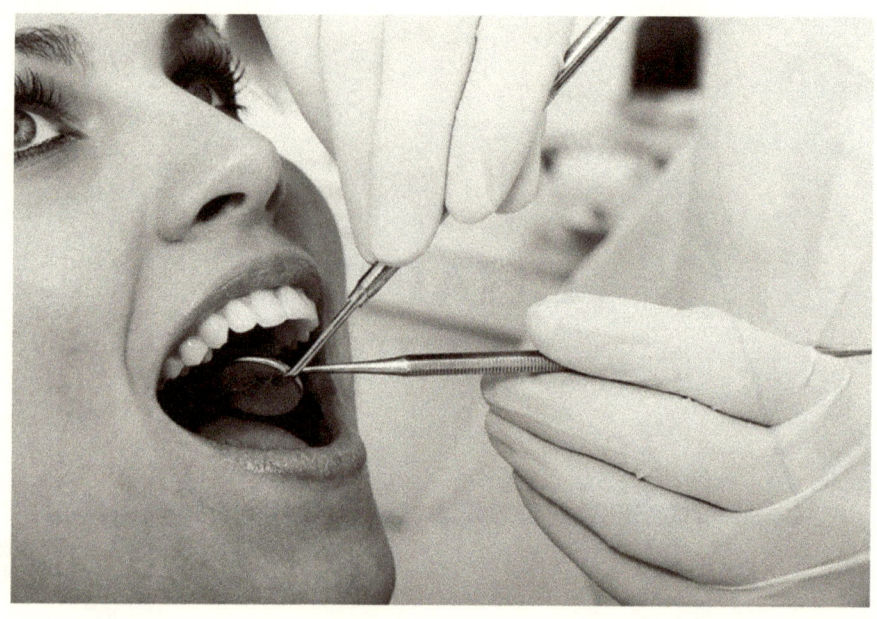

"Find a dentist, who is able to treat gaggers successfully."

WHY GAGGING IS A PROBLEM

In the Journal of the American Dental Association it was written: "Gagging in the dental office is a prevalent problem and dental care-related fear and fear of pain are associated with more frequent gagging." (JADA 145 (5) May 2014 pages 452-458)

TECHNIQUES AND "TRICKS" THAT WORK

Here are some of my techniques and "tricks" for patients with a gagging problem.

- ✓ Practice with your toothbrush weeks before your appointment, moving it further back in your mouth slightly each day until you can allow a dentist access without your gagging.
- ✓ Find a dentist, who is able to treat gaggers successfully.
- ✓ Ask your dentist to use nitrous oxide for your appointment.
- ✓ Ask for Non-IV Oral Conscious Sedation Dentistry using Triazolam.

TOOLS THAT CAN HELP

Here are some tools for gaggers to try (and suggest to their dentist).

- Ask for nitrous oxide for your dental treatment if you have a slight gagging issue.
- Locate a dentist that has taken a training course like DOCS Education and knows how to use Non-IV Oral Conscious Sedation using Triazolam.
- Try placing a teaspoon of kosher salt under your tongue before starting treatment.
- For impressions, you should speak with your dentist beforehand and ask if he or she is open to suggestions and will be amenable to the following steps for you.
    - Sit halfway up in the dental chair and practice having the dentist place in your mouth an unloaded impression tray until you have no gagging response. This may involve a separate appointment for you or you may be able to take an impression the same day.
    - Reassure yourself that you can do this while mentally preparing yourself.
    - When the impression is ready to be taken, ask your dentist to fill the tray as minimally as possible, using the fastest setting material.

- Suggest that your dentist place the tray starting from the back of your mouth to the front and remove all the excess immediately.

- Sit completely upright and lean all the way forward, (allowing yourself to drool, if necessary) and then focus on your legs while doing isometric leg and foot exercises, including lifts and stretches.

- You might feel like you are in an aerobics class and even somewhat foolish. However, I have helped numerous patients over the years with using only this technique.

- Try altering your gag reflex via a palm pressure point, located in the center of your palm. I suggest you first try this at home and see if it helps curb your gagging before trying it in the dental office. According to JADA, Vol. 139, October 2008, pages 1365-1372, "The gag reflex moves posteriorly toward the pharyngeal wall after application of pressure to this point."

HAVE NO FEAR OF THE DENTAL CHAIR!

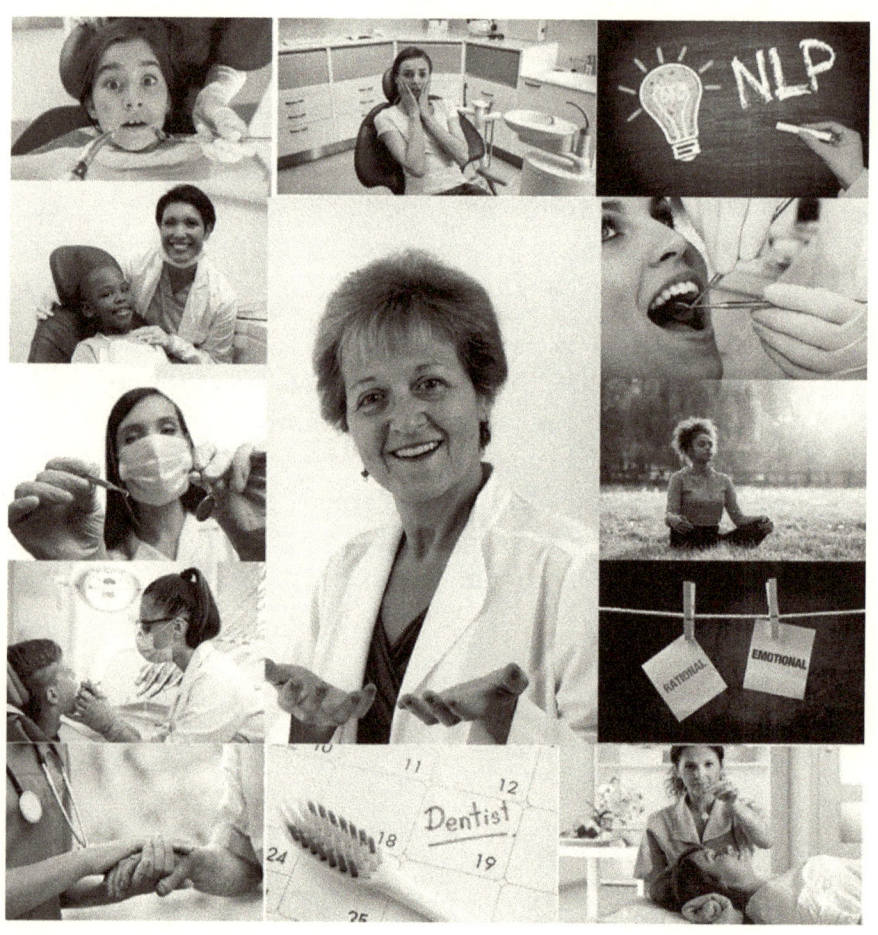

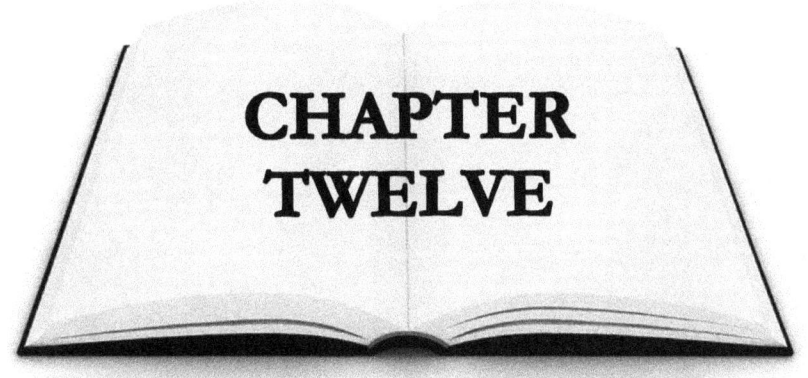

CHAPTER TWELVE

Childhood Dental Trauma
Simplest and Most Effective Tools Available

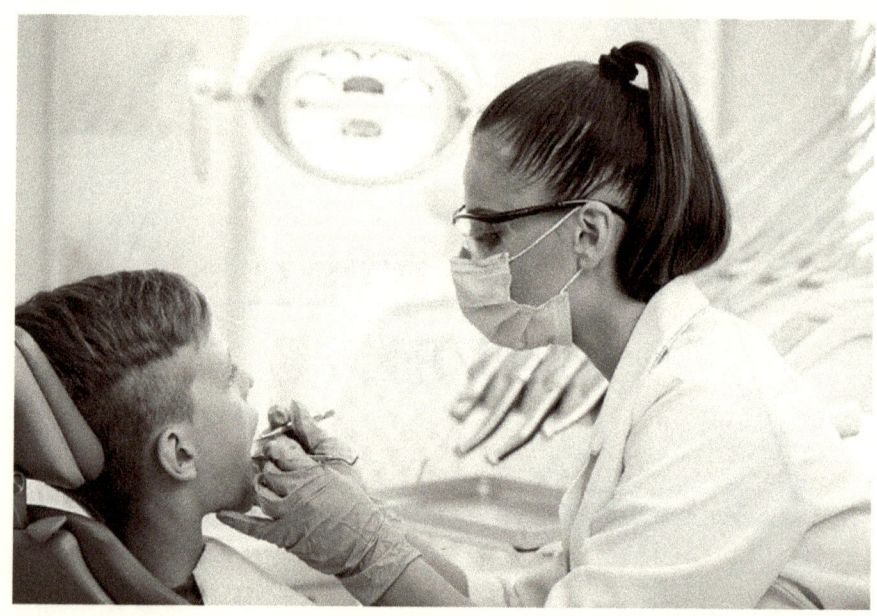

"An effective preventative behavior management technique for a child can begin with giving them a feeling of control."

CHILDHOOD DENTAL TRAUMA

One factor causing dental fear called "Iatrogenic Odontophobia" is under the control of the dental profession, according to an article in General Dentistry:

> "Iatrogenic Odontophobia is the dentist-instigated fear and phobia. Studies suggest that some if not a majority of dental phobics developed their problem as a result of dental care received as a child." (General dentistry, August 1991, *Undoing Iatrogenic Odontophobia*)

> "A composite statement from dental phobics might state: *When I was a child my dentist was rough, unpleasant, unkind, (He) hurt me, (He) abused me, (He) frightened me and (He) was mean to me.*"

What I have seen in my own experience is that for some people, just the thought of going to a dentist is so absolutely frightening that they put off treatment until they get an abscess or a severe toothache. By this time, however, there are usually only two options, removing the nerve (pulp) inside the tooth or removing (extracting) the tooth itself.

According to another article taken from General Dentistry (General Dentistry, Sept-Oct. 1995):

> "Patients with this degree of fear are called *Dental Phobics*. For many their fear originated in childhood, when they were hurt but were afraid to say anything so they wouldn't be yelled at. Some have reported that their hands and feet were held down or were intimidated aggressively to sit still and stop crying. It is also said that Dental phobia is an unnatural fear or an aversion to dentists and dental care."

I have also noticed that a majority of my adult patients with this type of fear have had negative childhood dental experiences. These unfortunate experiences had caused them to feel scared, threatened and unsafe as a child. Many have felt violated and powerless and decided at a young age to never return to the dental office willingly if possible (Just as I decided as a child after being hurt).

An effective preventative behavior management technique for a child can begin with giving them a feeling of control. Many Pediatric dentists or dentists specializing in treating only children, and many General Dentists use this valuable technique. Using the "show-tell-do" method works with the parent and child together on pre-treatment modeling and can offer the valuable technique of distraction.

SIMPLEST AND MOST EFFECTIVE TOOLS AVAILABLE

Here are the simplest and most effective "tools" available for both children and adults.

- ➤ A dentist that is kind.
- ➤ A dentist who has a truly genuine smile.
- ➤ A dentist who shows empathy for what the patient is experiencing and feeling.
- ➤ A dentist with a caring touch, when appropriate.
- ➤ Finding a dentist who talks directly to your child and establishes rapport.

> The child and parent both feeling they can trust the dentist.

> A dentist that listens to both the parent and the child and acknowledges that they heard, understood and believes what their patients are experiencing (validates their reality).

When you tell the dentist that you are feeling pain and are not numb, he or she should stop immediately and should not keep drilling. This is very important. It seems that too many dentists have done this over the years and told a patient: "I numbed you, you can't be feeling anything!"

AUTHOR NOTE: Here is a perfect example.

I recently treated a patient who was on "nitrous" and was still "jumpy". When I thought it might be more than his anxiety, I stopped and asked him what was going on.

He told me that he was feeling the drilling, but to keep drilling because he always felt the "drilling" at the dental office. I questioned him further and he shared with me that he has "never" been fully anesthetized during dental treatment and has been told each time he complains that: "You cannot be feeling this, you are numb."

He said that this situation had created a lot of anxiety for him since he was a child, but he eventually learned to sit as still as possible and hope the drilling stops quickly. He said that he wanted a healthy mouth and thought, "maybe it's all in my head and I am just crazy and the dentist is right."

I told him I did not want him feeling any pain if at all possible. I re-anesthetized him using additional anesthetic techniques, (various nerve blocks and infiltrations) and waited 15 minutes, giving extra time for the anesthetic to work.

Soon, he said he felt numb and asked me to try again. I successfully completed the restoration and watched him sit totally still throughout, breathing in the "nitrous" slow and steady.

When we were done he exclaimed in amazement: "I am 48 years old and this is the first time I have not felt any pain during the drilling. You're the first dentist that has ever fully numbed me. I have been thinking I was crazy for many years. Thank you."

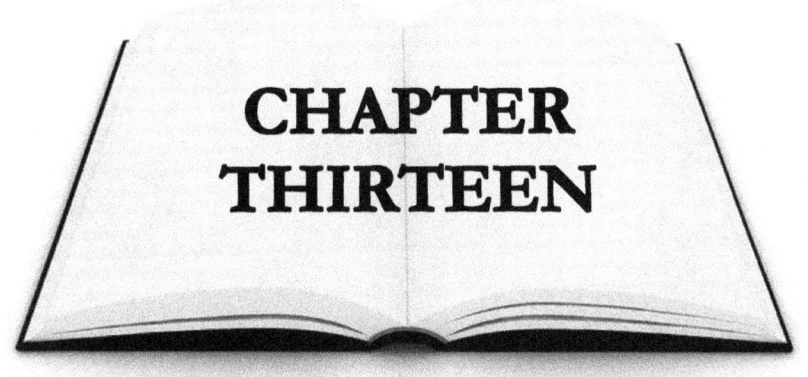

CHAPTER THIRTEEN

USING NEURO-LINGUISTIC PROGRAMMING (NLP) FOR DENTAL ANXIETY WITH THE PHOBIC PATIENT

"In Neuro-Linguistic Programming or NLP we are taught to calibrate or objectively notice, how a person is reacting and experiencing their present circumstance."

USING NLP FOR DENTAL ANXIETY WITH THE PHOBIC PATIENT

In Neuro-Linguistic Programming or NLP we are taught to calibrate or objectively notice, how a person is reacting and experiencing their present circumstance.

We want to determine what process or strategy a person's mind uses to function normally. There are processes called "V" (Visual), "A"(Auditory), "K"(Kinesthetic) and "In AD" (Internal Auditory Digital) going on in our minds constantly. The human mind is so quick and intelligent that it learns quickly. This can be extremely useful most of the time, but it can also have some drawbacks.

Here is an excellent example.

If a child goes to a dentist and gets hurt, (in whatever way that child perceives being hurt), that child experiences fear and will be careful not to get hurt again. If caught right away the fear may be able to be reduced by the dentist explaining the pain or an apology made. More often than not, both the child and the dentist can move past this single event and change the future to one where the child does not have the same experience.

However, if not caught or if it happens again, this same child has learned that going to a dentist is painful. He or she decides that a dentist cannot be trusted and is not a safe person. Then, all thoughts regarding a dentist in the child's memory are of pain and fear.

In addition, the child's nervous system has had a "traumatic" event and may store the pain experience neurologically to be recalled later whenever the need arises.

The child may have a Visual (V) memory of the dentist, seeing the needle or seeing other scary images; an Auditory (A) memory, hearing him or herself crying or screaming, yelling for their mother or hearing the drill; a Kinesthetic (K), memory of feeling the pain of the needle or drill; or an Internal Auditory Digital (In AD), memory), telling him or herself that because of the hurt suffered, the dentist is bad or other internal messages.

This learning stays buried in their subconscious mind for the rest of their lives and will come up again when something triggers it (sets it off). It could be when their mother says they have to go to the dentist, as in my case, or it could be many years later when they are an adult and experiencing a toothache. Either way, we now have a patient who has developed a dental anxiety or phobia and is in distress.

NLP has shown that no matter what we may say verbally or think we are communicating, our bodies are constantly giving away our real truths. We may say yes with our voice, while our head is actually shaking and signally "no."

AUTHOR'S NOTE: Actually, dear readers, it might be interesting for you to begin noticing yourselves and others for this fascinating phenomenon.

Most of us have heard that our body language is the majority of our communicating with the world. However, to experience it firsthand and learning how to use it effectively can be a real advantage in one's life.

An NLP practitioner who is skilled can help others by first determining what strategy or strategies the person uses and then guiding them to make safe and appropriate changes to benefit and improve themselves and their lives.

I determine a patient's strategy as follows:

1. Asking specific well-planned out questions (dental and non-dental), and "actively listening" to their responses including the actual language and intonations they use. If I am working with a patient, my questions concern their past dental experiences, present state and desired state or outcome; and

2. I carefully watch the patient's body language, facial movement, eye movements, color changes, moisture changes and twitches of hand and feet motions.

> **AUTHOR'S NOTE: A skilled NLP practitioner will be bombarded with input and take it all in as objective information without making any judgments or interpretation as to what it all means.**

3. Once I have determined what I believe is the patient's strategies, I confirm those strategies by testing them. When this is accomplished, I can help my patient figure out what he or she wants and how it can be achieved in very positive, clear and specific terms. Then, and only then, I offer an assortment of treatment modalities.

The goal is not to push my patients toward where they want to go. The goal is to guide them toward the result while encouraging them to trust their own "inner knowing" and what is best for them. It is a matter of meeting the patient where they are currently and helping them get to where they want to be in order to achieve the desired outcome.

Once the initial processes are completed and I have calibrated (noticed) that they have integrated and achieved their change in state congruently, I then guide them to imagine taking those resources to their near and distant future (future-pacing). This empowers them to carry these helpful changes into future situations and gives them more control.

One of the ways I do this is by adding in resources that the patient desires, but hasn't been able to obtain by themselves. It may be courage, trust, pleasure, joy, laughter or a sense of humor, confidence, feeling of safety, ability to have a voice and say no and the list goes on.

I achieve this by offering ideas, suggestions and strategies, (mental and physical). These physical resources I use are called kinesthetic anchors.

When I began doing this in my first dental office, I allotted ninety minutes per session. It was absolutely amazing to me to have a terrified, shaking patient, who was sweating and filled with fear, sit calmly and confidently at the end of their session. They usually share with me that they are not only "not afraid", but they do not remember ever being "that" afraid to begin with. To me it felt surreal! Some of my patients experienced life changing results in only one session. However, many require three to five sessions to achieve their goal. There were some patients who needed to go through the process very slowly due to their trust issues and others that could just jump right in. Many of those would see such a dramatic shift after only one session that they would request more sessions to work on other issues and personal limitations.

Interestingly enough, as effective and life altering as these NLP-AMC, (Anxiety Management Counseling) sessions could be, once Sedation Dentistry became an option, most of my patients decided they would rather just have sedation for their dental care.

I am extremely grateful that for many years I had the ability to offer NLP (AMC) when there was nothing else available.

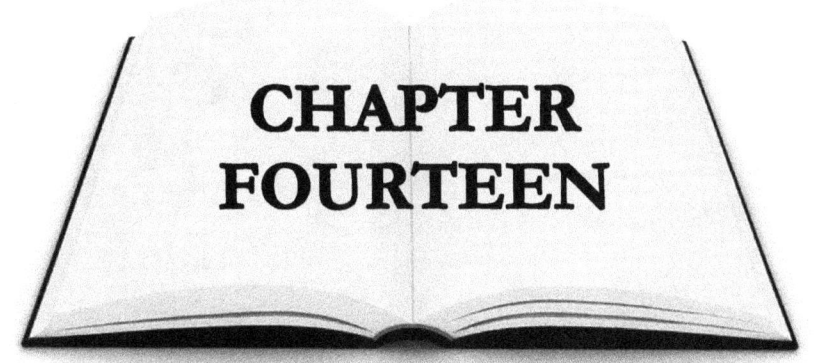

CHAPTER FOURTEEN

SELECTING THE TECHNIQUES THAT ARE BEST FOR YOU

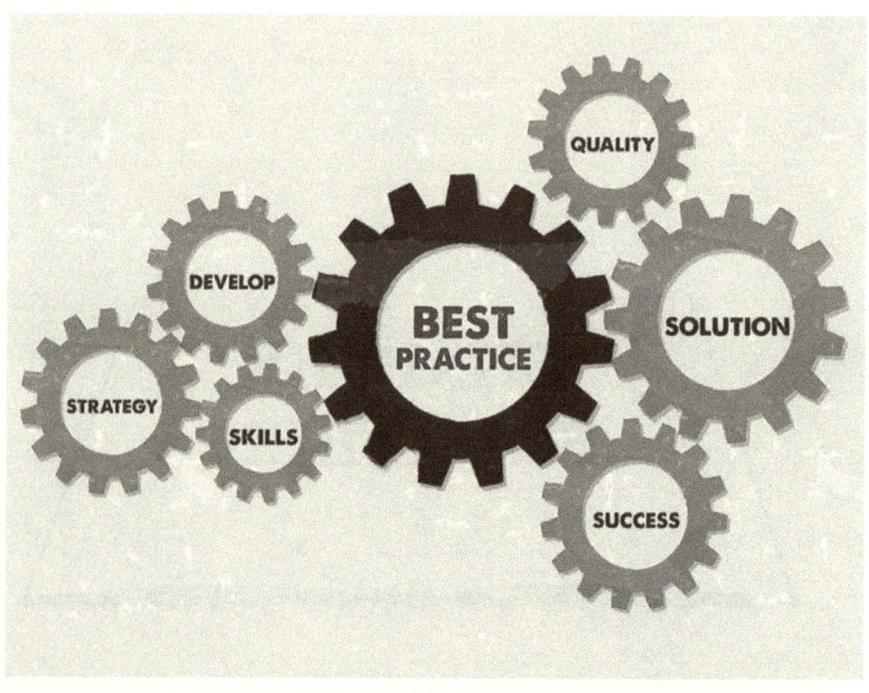

"In my opinion, in order to choose which techniques would be best for you, it is wise to consult with the dentist you have chosen after doing your research."

SELECTING THE BEST TECHNIQUES

In an article written in Access, April 1999 the following was stated: *"nitrous oxide, anti-anxiety agents such as Valium, and soothing music have long been available as methods of relieving anxiety, but there are also many more products using modern technology, like intra-oral cameras, relaxation tapes and patient viewing systems."*

In my opinion, in order to choose which technique or techniques would be best for you, you should consult with the dentist you have chosen. You might pick a dentist because of their particular skill or techniques. You might meet a dentist that you immediately connect with or feel like you can trust them to treat you the way you need to be treated. You might find an open-minded dentist willing to use one of the techniques or tools I have mentioned in order to help you with getting your dental care accomplished.

Ultimately, my advice to any fearful person is to choose a dentist and try the technique or techniques that seem to fit you best. If it does not give you what you expected or needed, then try another dentist or technique until you get your dental care accomplished without any anxiety or fear.

HAVE NO FEAR OF THE DENTAL CHAIR!

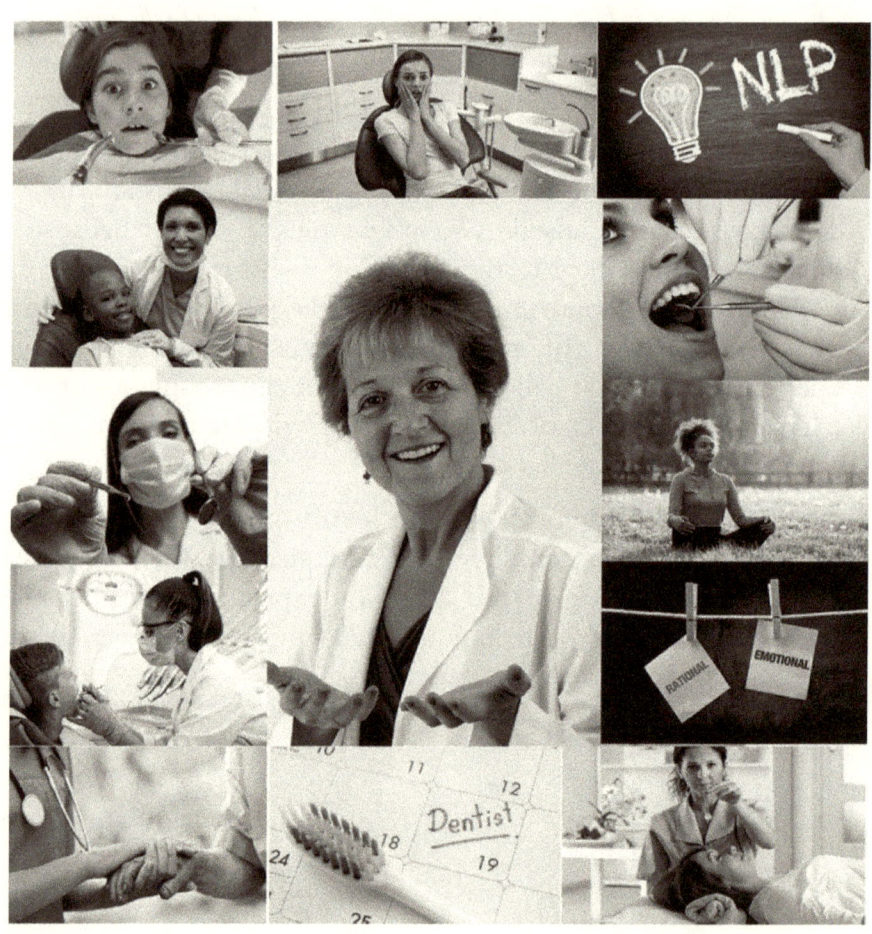

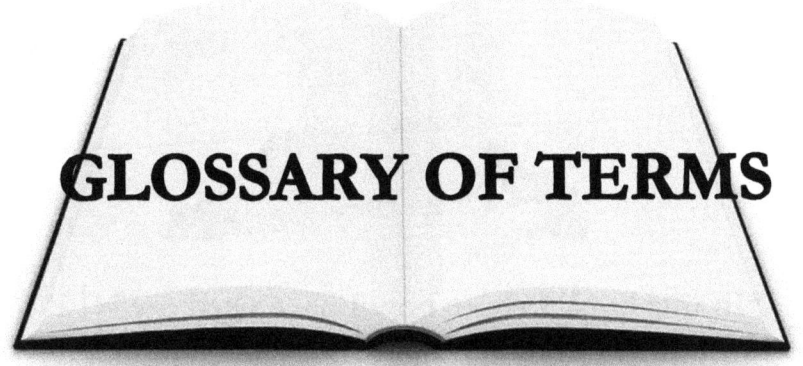

GLOSSARY OF TERMS

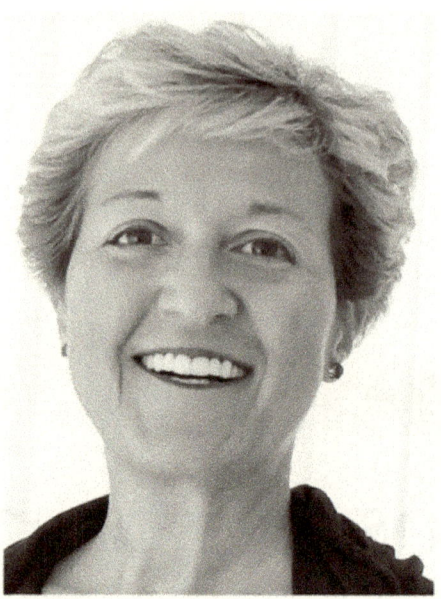

"In this book I share how I have used my NLP techniques to treat anxious patients and help them get over their dental anxiety and fears. In order to help you understand my process, I am including a glossary of terms relating to NLP and the dental terminology used."

GLOSSARY OF TERMS

AD or Auditory Digital - NLP term for the internal messages we think or the things we say to ourselves in our minds, our internal dialogues.

Anchor - The process of associating an internal response with some external or internal trigger so that the response can be accessed, an associative conditioning technique offering a stimulus and response, a physical cue that offers a specific behavioral action or feeling or causes you to behave in a certain way without your conscious awareness.

Anchors & Anchoring - Adding a connection to someone's repertoire that when triggered or set into use will bring to mind a memory or body sense (For example, if it is a visual anchor offering a visual component or picture to someone that will bring up a specific resource or memory for them, if it's a kinesthetic anchor-- it's an external touch that triggers an external event or causes you to feel a certain way).

Auditory & Auditory Channel - Internal channel for cognitive processing and interpretation of the world according to what we hear.

Back Pacing - A strategy the guide uses to understand, clarify and gain rapport with their client or patient, by repeating exactly what was said.

Calibrate - To objectively observe and measure another's body language, expressions, facial color and anything else that helps while you guide them during the NLP process. To closely watch the patient while noticing their body language, facial color, facial expressions and movement, their breathing, speaking pattern and any signs coming from them as the NLP Practitioner assesses them, works with them and guides them.

Calibrating - Closely observing another's external/physical communication. According to Jonathan Atfeld at Mastery Insight Institute, "In NLP-how well you "calibrate" to another person, and their state of mind, and what's going on inside their minds-determines to a significant degree how effective your communication will be with them."

Change Personal History - A process or intervention by which an NLP guide can help another person take the emotional power out of a past remembered event that has negatively affected them.

Crown - A tooth-shaped "cap" that is placed over a tooth to restore its shape, size and function.

Desensitize - To free someone from a phobia or neurosis by gradually exposing the person to the thing they feared, to make someone less likely to feel distress at a scene or of suffering by an overexposure to such images.

Dental Restoration or Dental Filling - A dental restorative material used to restore a tooth to health and function.

Desired Outcome - The end result of what a person or patient wants. In NLP, the guide or practitioner assists the patient to go from "where they are" to "where they want to go."

Desired State - The way a person wants to look like, sound like and feel like at the end of the session or process, what you want to achieve-as you visualize your outcome, using all five senses. This must be sensory specific.

Dentophobia - Fear of dentists.

Ecology - Assuring that the guide is working with the patients to protect them at all times and assuring that everything being done is in the patients best interests. During NLP processes asking the patient to go inward and confirming what is being worked on is helping that patient move forward safely.

EMDR - Eye movement desensitization and reprocessing- a psychotherapy treatment originally designed to alleviate the distress associated with traumatic memories, including symptoms of post-traumatic stress disorder.

First Position - This is the objective perspective of experiencing the world from the completely subjective perspective of the patient or person being guided (i.e. the one experiencing the situation). As if you were "standing in the person's shoes."

Future Pace - Guiding the patient to go into the future in their minds and imagining what it will be like for them using their newly anchored resource. This allows them to integrate it further, so it will be fully available to them when the time comes.

Future Pacing - Done at the end of an NLP process to ensure the changes received will be available to the patient after the patient leave the session.

Guide - Acting as the facilitator that helps another person access their inner thoughts, memories or strategies in order to reach a desired outcome.

Guiding - Helping another person access their inner thoughts, memories, strategies or ways of functioning using various NLP processes in order to reach a desired outcome for the better.

Infiltration - Injecting an anesthetic near the area a dentist wants anesthetized, usually only affecting the terminal branches of the nerves.

Install - To place an "anchor" or resource for a patient to access, in order to aid them in dealing with their fear or to help improve how they deal with an issue in their life.

Installing - The process of facilitating the gaining of a new strategy or behavior. A new strategy may be installed through some combination of anchoring, accessing cues, metaphor and future pacing.

Kinesthetic - Something externally felt, the cognitive processing and interpretation of the world according to what we feel and the emotions we experience in our body.

Milton Model Languaging - Can be described as hypnotic language used to help lead someone into a "zone" or "trance-like" state, a variety of persuasive and hypnotic languaging used to help a patient get into a more relaxed state of mind for the purpose of allowing the patient to have dental treatment performed and the treatment to flow smoothly.

Mirroring - The behavior where one person subconsciously (or consciously if done during NLP), imitates the gesture, speech pattern or attitude of another.

Nerve Block - Placement of the anesthetic adjacent to a major nerve or a major branch of the nerve that stops sensation from that point to the terminal end of the nerve.

NLP-Neuro-Linguistic Programming - An approach to communication, personal development and psychotherapy. According to Wikipedia: "a connection between the neurological processes ("Neuro"), language ("Linguistic") and behavioral patterns learned through experience ("Programming") and that these can be changed to achieve specific goals in life."

Odontophobia (also Dentophobia or Dental Phobia) – Refers to a fear of dentists or dental treatment, a condition depicting an irrational and overwhelming fear of dentistry, a fear of dental surgery, an abnormal fear of teeth-especially of animal teeth.

Operatory - The working space for the dentist, a room or other area with special equipment and facilities to do dentistry, the dental surgical suite or room where the dentist treats the patient.

Pacing and Leading - A strategy to respond just like the patient or person being guided to attain rapport. For example, when the patient talks you answer him back in the same tone and speed.

Patient's Map - Experiencing the world or situation and all that is happening from the mindset or perspective of the way a patient would view things. Remember, each patient is an individual, so each patient will view things differently depending on their life, past experiences, and all they have learned and gone through. It is as if the guide was actually inside the patients mind (rather than in their own mind), with access to all that this person has lived through, experienced seen, heard and felt and judged because of it. This is to help the guide fully understand where the patient is coming from and to be better able to guide the patient to a more useful outcome and what the patient would want.

Post and Core (occasionally referred to in an abbreviated form as a post) - A type of dental restoration used after a root canal is completed to stabilize a weakened tooth internally and provide an anchor for a crown.

Present State - The state of mind and body that one is starting out with, an identification of where a person is at with a particular problem or an assessment of their immediate present.

Pre-Suppositions - Suggesting an action to a patient that assumes a behavior they might do at the end of an NLP session or in the future (for the purpose of helping them live more effectively). These help to subtly direct a patient's future actions thru their unconscious in a gentle and positive manner.

Radiograph - An X-ray, taken to help diagnose dental problems.

Recare - A term used by the dental profession for ensuring regular, preventive dental treatment for their patients, regular 3, 4 or 6 months exam and cleaning appointments.

Resources - Character traits, assets, emotions and states of being that can be helpful to someone and make dealing with their difficulties better.

Reframing - Saying something in a different way to help offer a different and more useful perspective ("map of the world") to someone for the purpose of making them more resourceful.

Restoration - A dental restorative material to repair a damaged tooth, a dental restoration or a dental filling is a dental restorative material used to restore the shape, function and integrity of the missing tooth structure.

Root Canal or Endodontic Therapy - A dental procedure done to save a tooth by removing the diseased or injured nerve tissue in its root.

Second Position - Experiencing the world from the perspective of the one interacting with the person in a particular situation; the person relating to the patient or person being guided.

Third Position - Experiencing the world from the completely objective perspective of being an outside observer: as if from above the scene looking down on it or as if you "were a fly on the wall" with no judgment or hidden agenda.

Trigger (also referred to as the stimulus) - The automatic or unconscious mood change that occurs as a result of an external event that can cause us to take an action, what causes us to feel a certain way without any conscious awareness.

Visual - Something seen, the cognitive processing and interpretation of the world according to what we see in our minds while we are thinking.

Well-Formed Outcome - An outcome that a patient wants to achieve that meets specific measurable criteria. This goal must be integrated with all aspects of the person's life and has a process that respects and supports their current desirable circumstances.

HAVE NO FEAR OF THE DENTAL CHAIR!

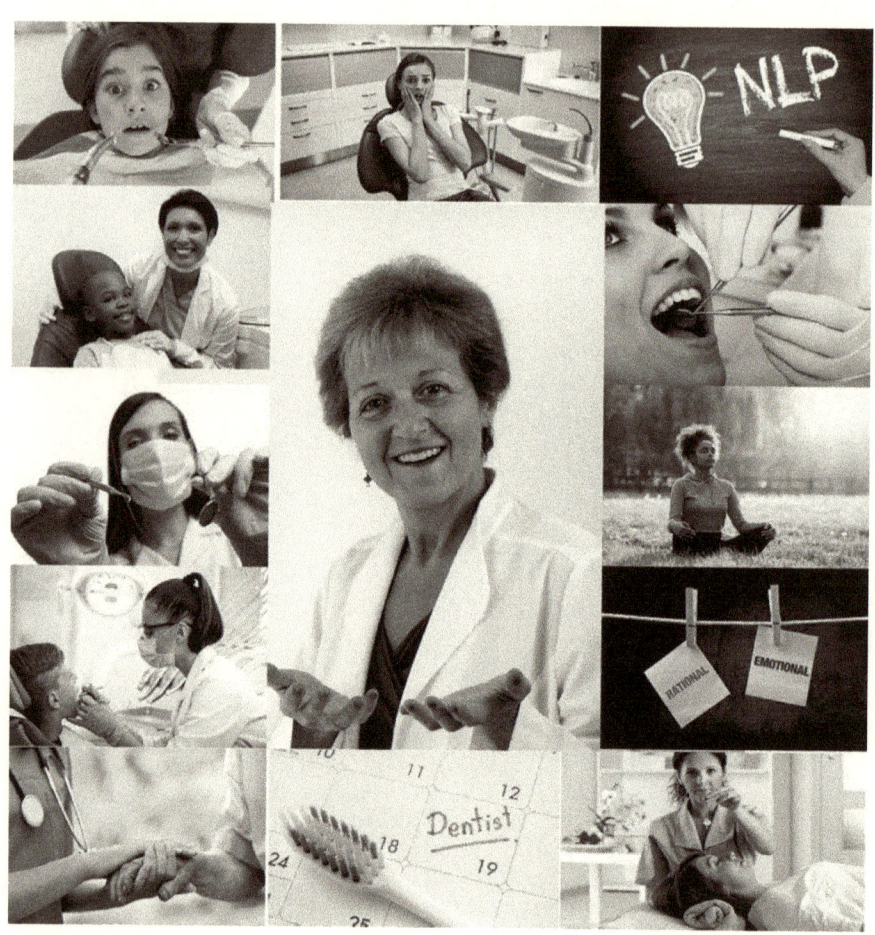

References

1. ADA Health Policy Institute. hpi@ada.org/ ext 2568, 145 (5) May 2014 pages 452-458, Gagging.

2. ADA Health Policy Institute unpublished 2014 findings from the Survey of Dental Practice (ADA News January 18, 2016, pages 1, 14).

3. American Dental Association (ADA) in April 1999. According to the article "Controlling Pain and Anxiety" by Caroline Bouffard, written in Access, April 1999, pages 14-18.

4. Dr. Arthur A. Weiner in the May 2002 AGD Impact Magazine.

5. JADA 146 (8), Aug 2015 (page 642).

6. ADA Survey center, 1997, Survey of Consumer Attitudes and Behavior Regarding Dental Issues.

7. Access, April 1999, page 17.

8. FDA report 2009 on Amalgam.

9. US Food and Drug Administration, Appendix I, July 28, 2009.

10. AAE, American Association of Endodontists, winter 2015 newsletter.

11. Lindagail and Associates, NLP Institute of Oregon, 1995.

12. The Journal of The Massachusetts Dental Society, winter 1999 magazine, page 9; "Using Mind-Body Techniques in Dentistry", by Eleanor F. Counselman, ED.D, ABPP.

13. Spiegel H, Spiegel D.; "Trance and Treatment"; Washington, DC: American Psychiatric Press; 1978).

14. Glamour Magazine, April 1988, pages 72-78.

15. AGD Impact Magazine, July 1994, pages 9-11.

16. AGD Impact Magazine, October 1993, page 14.

17. JADA 145 (3), page 240.

18. Time Magazine April 2, 2001, pages 50-62; "What Scares You?"

19. General Dentistry, May-June 1994, page 237.

20. JADA 145 (3), page 238.

21. AGD Impact Magazine, Dental Fact Sheet on Dental Anxiety, February 2015.

22. Romeo Vitelli, Ph.D. (Psychology Today, Media Spotlight, Staying in Control, posted October 21, 2013).

23. JADA 145 (5) May 2014, pages 452-458.

24. JADA, Vol. 139, October 2008, pages 1365-1372.

25. General Dentistry, August 1991, "Undoing Iatrogenic Odontophobia."

26. General Dentistry, Sept-Oct. 1995.

27. AGD Impact Magazine, April 1999, page 19.

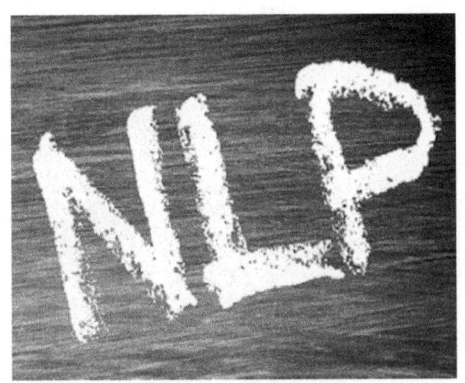

NINETEEN NLP CASES AND TWO INTERESTING STORIES

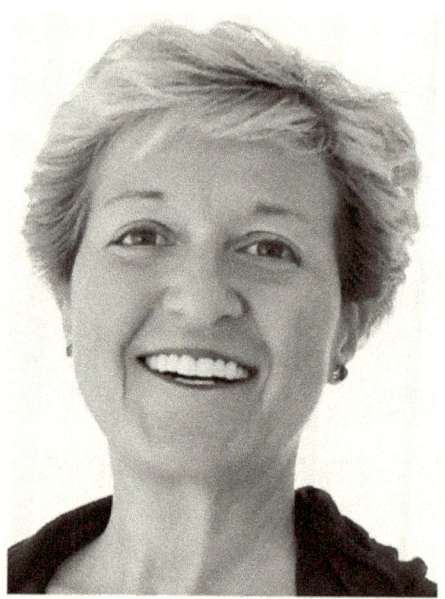

"To show what is actually possible using NLP, here are some of my most interesting patient experiences. As you read each one, see if you can identify with any of them. If you are especially fearful or call yourself a dental phobic, consider if any technique used here could work for you or someone you know."

CASE #1

[Note-This was one of my more challenging and complicated cases.]

JS arrived to my office appearing very quiet and reserved. She filled out her paperwork as instructed and then my assistant brought her back to one of my operatories. While taking her radiographs (X-Rays), my assistant noticed how frightened she was, stopped and quickly got me.

I came into the room and sat down beside JS and noticed just how frozen she looked. Her whole body was tense and tight and her neck appeared rigid. She was clasping her hands together and releasing them over and over and when I went to shake her right hand, it felt moist and clammy.

As I visited with her, tears flowed down her face and although she had at first appeared in control, she began to cry uncontrollably saying, "This is so silly, I shouldn't be so afraid".

I validated her feelings, obtained rapport and shared with her some of my dental history and personal story of intense dental fear. As I did so, I added in presuppositions of how I could help her and related some stories of other fearful patients and how I had helped them.

I calibrated that although JS was trying to listen to me, she was too anxious to actually focus and take much of it in. By pacing and leading I was able to get a little of her dental background, but it was just too traumatic for her. I decided that the best way that I could help her was to schedule an NLP-AMC private session.

I described NLP and how the appointment would go and she was amenable to trying it. She said, "My main goal is to get over my fear of dentists. I feel so silly about this, but I just die for days ahead just thinking about it. I make an appointment a few weeks ahead and then I cancel it right before." She said that she couldn't imagine how the NLP would help, but she was ready to try just about anything.

At the end of this interview, JS had stopped crying. However, she still seemed "off balance and shaky" to me. I acknowledged her for coming in, validated what courage it took to enter a dental office considering her anxiety level and walked her to the front desk to schedule her NLP appointment.

She was still so unnerved, that I suggested that she take a seat in the reception area to relax for a bit and leave when she felt good enough to drive home. I also offered to have one of my staff take her home, but she declined. I told her to relax and I would call her later to make the appointment.

She seemed relieved and welcomed the suggestion. When I called her a few hours later, I congratulated her on actually coming to my office and asked how she was doing. She thanked me and asked if she could come in as soon as possible, before she became too terrified again. I scheduled her the following afternoon to begin the NLP process and she thanked me for getting her in so quickly.

The next day when she came in she still appeared afraid and yet she shared with me that she was somewhat curious about this NLP process and was "more than ready" to get over her dental fear. I re-introduced her to my dental assistant and asked if it would be okay for my assistant to take a full series of dental radiographs. I knew this would be an easy dental treatment that would help her begin to become desensitized to us working in her mouth and comfortable with our office and equipment. She agreed and did quite well.

My assistant brought her into my consultation room and I began strengthening my rapport with her. I knew from our last encounter that asking her right away about her dental history might stir up more than she could handle, so I began by working with her to get a well-formed outcome. She told me once again that she wanted to "not be afraid anymore." In NLP we want to have the desired outcome stated in positive terms and for the patient to be as specific as possible. My job as her guide was to pace and lead her until she could do that.

She finally came up with the following desired outcome, "I want to be fearless, I want to have trust that you won't hurt me or lie to me, know that I'll be safe and comfortable, and most of all I want to be relaxed throughout my entire body." She said that she considered picking courage, but decided that she already had courage since she had made it to our office two times. So, she decided to choose being fearless.

I checked her ecology thoroughly and found it solid and safe to proceed. Whenever I do NLP with my phobic patients, I like to start by explaining what process I will be doing before I proceed, in order to increase their trust in me and prepare them to participate in their own healing work.

During her process, I asked her to consider a comparable situation where she had all the positive resources that she said she wanted for her dental care. She very quickly told me it was with her Acupuncturist. So, I set a strong anchor kinesthetically (physically) on her right hand using this resource, a location that we would both have full access to for the rest of our session as the need arose. I call this a "safety" resource anchor.

I next prepared JS for the NLP "Phobia Removal" process using an imagined movie screen in a theater. I asked her to use one of her past childhood, traumatic dental experiences and reassured her that I would be helping her to feel safe the entire time. She stated that it was difficult because "they all are stuck together". I let her know that would work just fine, and suggested that she try "allowing her unconscious mind" to sort through her memories and choose the most vivid one if possible and to trust it would be the perfect one.

I guided her to run the memory like a black & white movie going forward as slowly as possible letting her "other than conscious mind" watch closely and learn from the scene and notice anything she wasn't already aware of that might help her. As I talked with her, I triggered (touched and held onto) her "safety" resource anchor all the while calibrating her ecology and body responses.

I also reminded her that she was "only watching a movie" from a very "distant and safe place" through a thick Plexiglas screen in a projection room. I told her the Plexiglas screen could get wider or thinner as she deemed necessary for her safety and optimum protection.

When I calibrated that she was ready, I asked her to run the same movie backwards as fast as she could and in full color going from a safe ending point to a safe beginning point. I directed her to do this 3 times and when I noticed that her eyes were still tearing up, I asked her to keep running it backwards a few more times.

I then had her run the movie in segments both forward and backwards until I saw that she no longer had tears running down her cheeks, that her face appeared more relaxed and that her body was slouching slightly in the chair.

When I calibrated that the process for her was complete, I tested her results by asking: "How do you experience that same situation now as you think about it?"

She began to look up and to her left (an NLP sign that she was going back in time in her mind), and then she said: "It's better, but still terrible. That dentist was a monster," and she began to cry again. She related the story behind the event as tears flowed freely down her face and she was breathing heavily. As I guided her back to our current moment, I held onto her safety anchor and watched as she slowly pulled herself out of the negative state and she began to share with me the implications and consequences of the incident that she gleamed from watching the movie.

As with many repressed memories there were other people involved and other events that she had not been able to remember before. She said she was surprised that she could even remember the complete event and be able to talk about it as calmly as she was. I told her that showed the process was working; now that she had remembered the incident she could access it and deal with it.

I determined we now needed to do the "Change Personal History" process and have her run a new movie of the event where she could give the others in the scene the resources that would change the event to how she would have wanted it to be.

She proceeded without hesitation and became quite involved in running her new movie. I directed her to add in whatever she needed to and to remember anything she might want to share with me later.

Soon her hands had stopped sweating, were lying calmly on her lap instead of being clasped on and off, her breathing was more even and not heavy or barely visible and she appeared much more relaxed. I noted that the coloring of her face and hands were more natural and pink instead of pale and flushed.

She told me she wanted to tell me what she had done to feel better and I was curious and prepared to find out what had made such a difference. She said that she had "disappeared the dentist and put in someone she liked and cared about and made a few other changes and the scene was much better." We discussed her learnings and how we could incorporate them into her appointments with me.

As she considered this I retested her anchor and determined that it had lost some of its previous strength, so with her permission, I asked her to close her eyes and we added in more "juicy and powerful" positive anchors that she had gained from the last process. I noticed that she, like most of the people I worked with, did much better when their eyes were closed. I re-tested her anchor again and both of us agreed that she was now ready to continue the process.

Next, I helped to transfer her strengthened, powerful anchor onto a place that she chose on her left finger, so that she could have total access while sitting in the dental office or for anytime she decided to use it. (I had decided to offer this anchor- position transfer early on in my practice of NLP, in order to help my patients improve their lives inside of and outside of my office.)

I then did additional testing and future pacing to insure that we had completed the goals for her session. I reviewed with her that she now had a personal anchor that she could use in my office or at any time she wanted her powerful resource available.

Lastly, I gave her some assignments that would add to her NLP experience and to help her prepare for her upcoming dental appointment.

She was smiling full face for the first time since I had met her and she kept telling me how much better she felt and how pleased she was. I asked her if there was anything left that she felt she still needed before leaving. She closed her eyes and suddenly jumped up in her chair, eyes wide open and said, "Yes! Is there anything major that will happen in my mouth before my next appointment? I have a diving trip planned next week and am worried that I'll have pain when I dive." Calibrating her anxiety starting again and knowing that she already had spent enough time in my office that day, I paced and led her to relax and then I reviewed her radiographs. The x-rays showed that there were no serious dental issues that should blow up in the next few weeks to cause her distress, so I acknowledged her fear and reassured her that she could go on her diving trip with confidence and when she returned I would do a comprehensive exam and develop her treatment plan.

She immediately resumed her smile and said: "That was one of my biggest worries, but I trust you and believe the preparation we did today will help me when I return, so I won't worry." She also told me that she wanted to start meditating and she could tell that the processes and visualization we had just done would help her. She thanked me, hugged me, scheduled her next dental appointment and left. As I watched her leaving, I calibrated what I would call a satisfied smile on her face, a relaxed body movement and lightness in her step.

When JS returned to my office four weeks later, we made full use of her personal anchor and the one I had access to and she did beautifully.

HAVE NO FEAR OF THE DENTAL CHAIR!

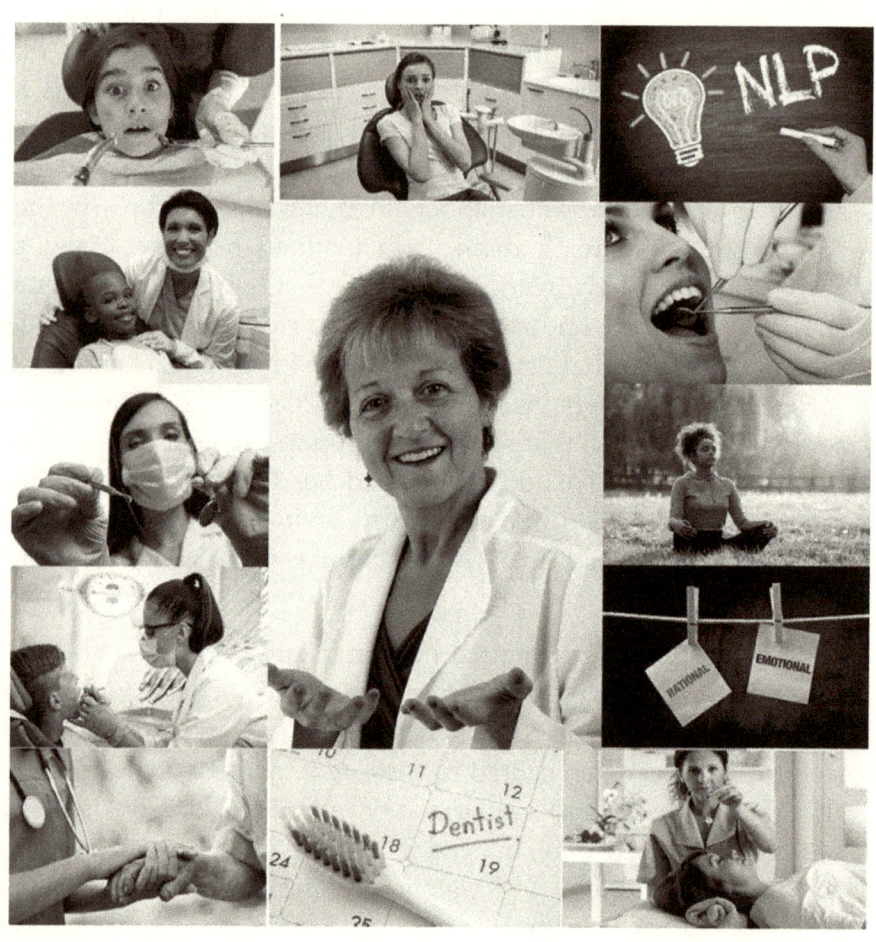

CASE #2

SD came to me saying: "I want to be able to get all my front crowns done and be proud of my smile." Her greatest fear was having any dental impressions taken because she "panics and then gags."

She told me that she had had a bad experience while in the Military in 1985; "When the upper impression was taken I began to gag and panic. I was shaking and couldn't swallow. The dentist got extremely frustrated and angry with me." She said she went back and tried it again, but was unsuccessful and gave up. "From that time on anything that goes too far back in my throat makes me gag, even my toothbrush."

SD's desire was "I want to have control and be able to express my needs, have them respected and get my front teeth fixed without gagging."

In her NLP session, I guided her via visualization and helped give her some desired resources and a safety anchor, which I placed kinesthetically (physically) on her arm. Then, while "triggering" this positive anchor (holding it and setting it off) I had her imagine being in a movie theater, sitting in the audience and running the entire experience while noticing it all from a safe distance away.

Then, I had her run her movie backwards and forwards and mix up all the segments over and over until she told me she felt comfortable watching it. I then asked her to use her inner resource of "control" and notice what she wanted to change in the movie and gave her time to do so. She took quite a bit of time to tweak it exactly as she wanted it to be. When she assured me all the changes had been made to her satisfaction and she was ready to move on, I tested it by having her run the movie once more.

This time she had no outward signs of anxiety or panic and actually looked somewhat peaceful. I had her imagine what her next appointment might be like using what she had just learned from the experience (future-pace). She did so as I watched her relax further in the chair and saw her entire face "soften" and appear "calm". When this NLP-AMC session was over, she said she had what she needed, felt comfortable and wanted to proceed right away.

I began by retesting her newly established anchor, just to be sure and began by placing various size impression trays in her mouth small ones at first and when she did well with those, I tried some larger ones we would need for her actual dental treatment. I gave her some time to practice and "desensitize" herself and gain confidence while I guided her and watched closely. Then I gave her the impression trays we would be using at the next appointment and assigned her "homework" telling her to practice with them at home.

She returned in one week saying she was completely ready and could even brush her back teeth now without gagging. We were able to take the preliminary impressions for her temporary crowns and do crown preparations of her front teeth including the final impressions with NO incident of gagging.

When she returned a few weeks later to cement her final crowns, she shared with me just how grateful she was to have found me and to finally resolve her long standing problem.

HAVE NO FEAR OF THE DENTAL CHAIR!

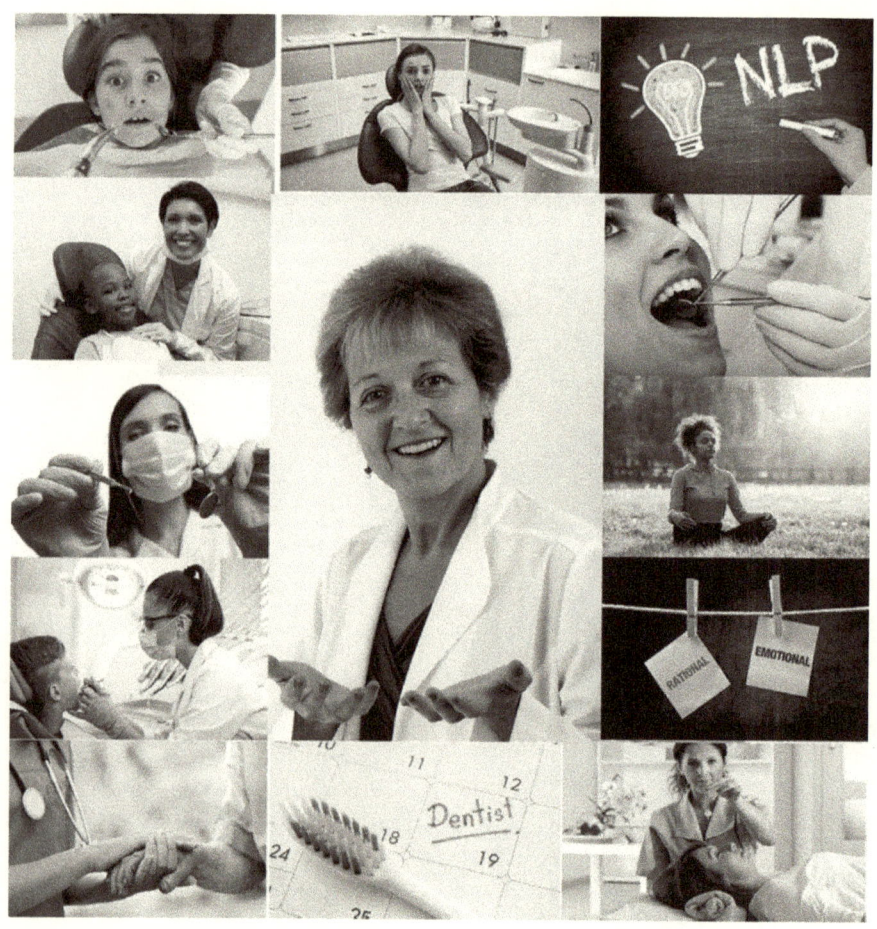

CASE #3

AP came in for a consult only to meet me and decide if she liked me. She told me she had gone to Dr. P. in town, but found her "cold and insensitive." She told me that she needs to know what is going on during treatment and has to stop during her appointments to have one of her many "props."

This patient carried a grocery sack full of items, including juice, crackers, aspirin, Tums, raisins, bottled water, a radio with headphones and much more that she chose not to discuss with me. She shared with me that she had quit smoking a year before and had gained a lot of weight that increased her blood sugar levels, which made her sick. Then she said: "I got sick in the head".

Her goal was twofold. She wanted to be able to sit still and get her dental treatment done and she wanted to get some needed blood work done. She had to have gall bladder surgery, but had been unable to get the required pre-testing blood work. She said that she was afraid of the unknown and kept cancelling appointments.

AP said she had heard about my Anxiety Management Counseling (NLP-AMC) sessions and felt she would be better able to handle any stressful situation, including her medical and dental appointments after NLP, so she decided to schedule her first session in two weeks.

When she returned she carried her grocery bag of "props" and kept it close to her. She appeared agitated and restless and was unable to sit still. She said she "hates bright lights." So, all the overhead lights in my private consultation room were dimmed.

She shared that she had been ill all winter and being sick makes me angry. She said that she "went crazy this winter from so much stress and began to have panic attacks just like the ones I had in childhood." She said that her father used to tell her "anticipation is worse than participation." She related that her mother was an alcoholic and she chose to live with her as a caretaker for the last four years of her mother's life where she had to "dose her drugs." She also told me that when she was six years old her sister died and that had traumatized her father so much that he began taking AP to the doctor for any real or imagined ailment.

Her ultimate goal was to get the necessary blood tests including her two hour IV pre-surgical test so she could have her gall bladder surgery. She also wanted to be able to sit still in a dental chair and get her treatment done.

When I began her NLP session, she discussed her anxieties and fear of "the unknown". I guided her to imagine what she needed to feel safe and when she did so, she was able to come up with an "action plan" to turn "the unknown" lab and hospital appointments into "knowns."

I asked her to decide what resources she needed and when she did, I helped "install" them using anchors, both physical (kinesthetic) and verbal (auditory). I arranged her physical anchor on her left hand so that it was fully available to her as she needed it. I also added in positive suggestions and ways she could take care of herself in addition to and possibly instead of all her "props," when she was ready to let them go.

I calibrated her shift in state and tested the results. At the end of our session I allowed her time to process her current state and to review whatever else she felt she needed. She said she felt like she was all set and ready to schedule a dental treatment appointment.

AP returned three weeks later for her dental appointment. She carried with her a shopping bag, but this time all she had inside was a bottle of water, a box of raisins and a radio with a pair of headsets. She told me that she had gotten the required blood tests and had completed her two hour pre-surgical IV test, and she had a date scheduled for her gall bladder surgery. She told me that she felt fully prepared and ready for her dental treatment that day. The dental procedure that day went reasonably well and at the end she thanked me for all I had done to get her to that point.

HAVE NO FEAR OF THE DENTAL CHAIR!

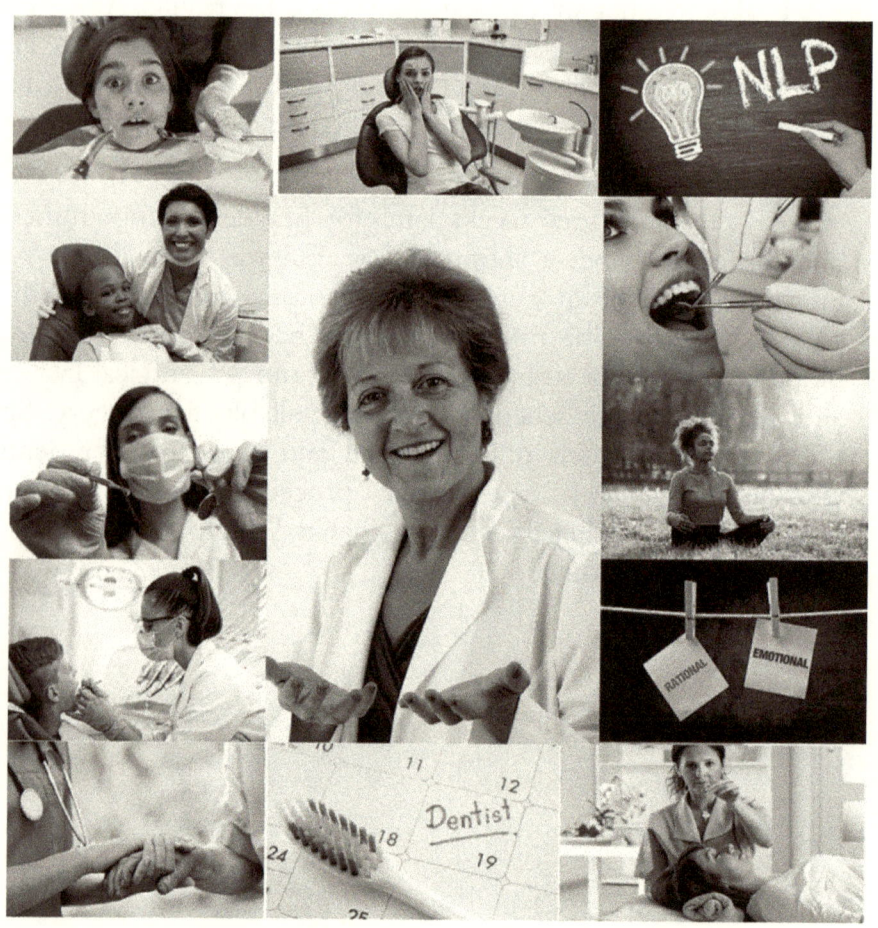

CASE #4

PC arrived to my office with the Chief Concern, (CC), "I have a lot of dental anxiety and the waiting makes me so anxious I can't stand it, so I never go." She said that her anxiety begins one week before her dental appointments when she feels "fearful, nauseous and out of control."

She told me that she had her first dental visit at age eight and the next one at age seventeen when she had a severe toothache. The appointment was "very traumatic." She said: "The dentist was rough and abrupt". Then, at age twenty-three she went for a cleaning and felt "tense waiting in the waiting room". The next five years she spent trying one dentist after another, but couldn't find one she was comfortable with. Then, at age twenty-eight, she needed to have her wisdom teeth removed and went to a dentist she was referred to. She said that her procedure went well, but when she stood up to leave the room she fainted, "I remember the dentist got angry, grabbed my arm and yelled at me." So, she waited another few years and found Dr. L. "He was elderly, very gentle and very small and I was comfortable with him for eight years." Then, she moved to Boise and was now at my office. She said, "Here I am once again extremely apprehensive and anxious and need some help."

I spent her NLP session learning what she wanted for her desired outcome by actively listening and guiding her through some visualization. Once I knew what "resources" she needed to make her comfortable at the dental appointment, I "anchored" them, (placed them physically on her arm), for her.

The "resources" she desired was "feeling peaceful, picturing myself being comfortable before, during and after my appointment and leaving happy and okay."

At the end of our session she looked visibly changed and ready for her appointment the following day. She assured me that she knew that she had gotten what she wanted. Just to be sure, I tested her anchor, as I always do, and her anchor worked well.

When she returned the following day, we practiced her anchor before I started any dental treatment and she responded beautifully. The appointment went smoothly and at the end she thanked me for treating her so well. She said, "I feel more confident in myself for my future visits. I know I will be just fine."

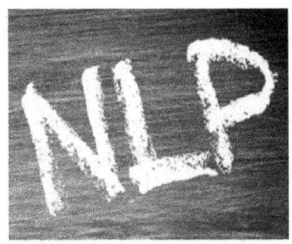

CASE #5

LW arrived to my office saying that her greatest fear is "pain" and her panic begins when she is in the dental chair. As she talked about her crying in the reception area when she was sixteen years old, I noticed that her hands were clenching and tightening continuously. When she related her bad experience five years before in Seattle when the dentist was "rough" during a cleaning and how her gums bled for a month after, I watched her cower in the chair and begin fidgeting seeming to be unable to get comfortable in her seat. She said she had a fear of the unknown and when she thinks of getting her teeth drilled and filled, she "can barely stand the stress."

She said her desire was to "feel more peaceful with a sense of security during dental treatment."

I asked her to share with me what resources she thought she would need in order to reach her goal. After she did so, I physically anchored those positive resources on her right arm and tested the anchor to be sure it was strong enough. When I was confident she had a strong anchor, I asked her to visualize what one of her bad experiences was like. I held onto her resource anchor and watched as her body began shivering all over and she rocked in her seat from front to back and then from side to side. After a few minutes, her body stopped moving and she became still and appeared to be completely relaxed. I checked in with her and she said that she felt calmer.

Next, I had her imagine what she wanted at that moment and what she would like her dental experience to be like. I told her to keep that thought forefront in her mind while she did the next process of running a movie. I used the model of the movie theater that allowed her to safely experience and watch her movie, seeing her past. During this process, I firmly held onto her resource anchor. I asked her to make the changes she desired, view it again, and to keep tweaking it until she was completely satisfied that the new desired scenario was what she wanted. I tested it and helped her be sure she had it solidly in place. Then, we "future paced" the desired outcome she wanted and had her view how she would handle herself at future dental appointments. As she did this, I closely calibrated to confirm that she had achieved exactly what she said she wanted and was ready to leave my office. When we were done, AP told me she could not believe how excited she was to return to my dental office and start her dentistry.

At her next dental appointment, I reviewed the treatment that was planned, tested her anchor and state of being and proceeded with her treatment. I talked to her throughout the appointment as she had requested, using verbal reassurances as discussed at her NLP-AMC session. She reassured me that she felt safe and in control. LW did extremely well throughout her appointment and said she felt wonderful at the end.

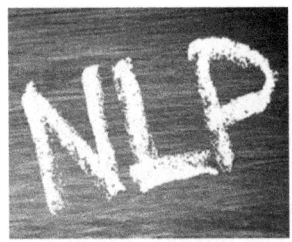

CASE #6

KG arrived to her NLP session saying, "I am extremely fearful of pain." She shared that for many years she told herself that she needed to go to the dentist to finish up the work that was started a long time ago. However, as soon as she remembers that when she was eight years old the dentist cut the side of her mouth with a bur, and there was so much blood she couldn't stand it, she decides that she "cannot go on." She told me that she has scheduled many dental appointments to get her work done, but as soon as she gets to the dental office, she cannot go any further and leaves.

As she talked about her past experiences, she remembered that she always had difficulty getting numb and had felt pain more than once during dental treatment. She said that she was afraid of nitrous oxide, because she gets nauseated easily and it happened one time as a child. She said that she gets so wound up during any dental appointment that she leaves totally exhausted and cannot drive herself home. She also remembered reacting to getting anesthetic one time where she actually fainted and then felt embarrassed.

KG said her goal was "to get my dentistry completed." She stated quite firmly, "I have to know what is being done and exactly how long I'll be in the chair. I need to start with a short appointment as a test, feel absolutely no pain at any time, and I want to feel a sense of accomplishment at the end instead of feeling like a failure."

As I considered her needs and what might suit her best, I determined that the best process for her would be to create a strong safety anchor filled with many positive resources. When I asked her what specific attributes would help her accomplish her goals she seemed to go blank. Since I could see that she was having difficulty accessing what resources she could draw on, I had her imagine what she respected and wanted from others she admired. Within a few minutes, she was able to come up with some resources that she believed was exactly what she needed. After creating her anchor and installing it on her right forearm, I guided her through a visualization of her upcoming dental appointment, where she would be using her new resources. We tested and future paced until she looked fully relaxed, engaged, and confident. Once she realized that her anchor worked, she told me she was ready to schedule her first treatment appointment.

She returned in three days for her short "test" appointment for one extraction and did extremely well. At the end, she said that she felt "at peace within herself and a true success and ready to move forward" and wanted to continue as soon as possible.

We were able to complete all of her restorative treatment comfortably in only a few appointments.

CASE #7

DS came into my consult room and shared with me that his greatest fear was of needles. He said that it started at about age three or four years old when he was running with a pen in his mouth, fell down and the pen pushed thru his uvula and into the back of his throat causing extensive damage. His mother took him to the emergency room and had to "hold him down while they repaired the damage."

He remembers being afraid of vaccinations and all needles. He told me that when he was ten years old and scheduled for an eye appointment, his older brother terrorized him by telling him that the doctor was going to stick a needle in his eye. He said that he worried about that for days and all through his eye exam.

He told me that he anticipates pain ahead of time and it builds up in his mind. Then when he gets to a dental appointment, he is so afraid that the dentist will start drilling before he is fully numb, that he shakes and won't open up his mouth to allow the needle in to get him numb.

I asked him a lot of questions in order to learn what might help him feel safe and comfortable and found out it was his three cats. So, I helped anchor his resource of feeling safe and comfortable while his favorite cat, Ben, was sitting on his chest purring. Using a visualization process, I trained DS to focus on

Ben's purring whenever he thought he felt the needle or became afraid of pain. We did some additional processes and soon DS was able to bypass any negative feelings of fear in his visualization.

I reassured him that he could ask for a rest break at any time during his treatment, which he had complete control over and could ask for what he needed. I also reviewed the communication signal for when he needed me to stop. After telling him this, he surprised me when he abruptly sat upright in his chair and told me that he had just remembered some past traumas. He then said, "I feel differently now. I know I don't have to just lay there and be stupid."

He told me that he felt ready to schedule an appointment to get his work done. As I looked at his expressive face, I calibrated that he had lost the dark, splotchy, red coloring in his face, that had appeared as soon as he began the visualization of his past traumas and fear of needles. I noted that his face had resumed its natural color and I could see that his body was congruent with his words. I tested his anchor to be sure the resources were fully available to him and seeing that they were, I future paced him and scheduled a dental appointment two days later.

When he returned, DS appeared much calmer and said, "I am ready to go." The treatment went well and he did extremely well. At the end of his appointment, DS said to me "That was better than I could have ever expected, thanks."

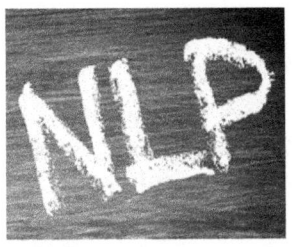

CASE #8

SS was not overly anxious when she came to my office. When I introduced myself to her, she said, "This is the year to get my mouth completely fixed." She was quite forthright when she told me, "I need to be heard and know that I'll get everything I need to keep me safe, comfortable and not hurt." She told me that in the past she has trusted dentists, then they hurt her and she would feel betrayed, so she stopped going for a period of time.

Her desire was to "feel mellow with a peaceful sense of fulfillment." She told me that she wants to be free to express her needs, have no surprises and be made aware of everything being done. I discussed with her what anxiety reducing options I offered and she told me that she had been referred from friends she fully trusted, felt very comfortable with me and felt like she could trust me. She said she really didn't need any NLP-AMC sessions and wanted to just have the nitrous oxide and use headphones. I agreed with her decision and scheduled her for the following Monday.

On Monday, she arrived thirty minutes early as planned. I placed her on oxygen, for a few minutes, and began the nitrous oxide at 30% and still seeing anxiety. Then, I increased it to 40%. My assistant placed the topical anesthetic and I fully anesthetized her upper left and lower left quadrants (1/2 of her mouth). We had her put on her headphones and turn on her CD player and let her listen to her music for 20 minutes while the anesthetic took effect. We covered her in the special blanket she had brought with her while we prepared for the restorative treatment. When she said, "I'm in la-la land and am happy and relaxed" as the sign agreed on at her consult appointment, I began her dental treatment.

SS did extremely well during the treatment and after flushing her with oxygen for ten minutes we had her rest in the chair until she was back to her normal state. She scheduled her next appointment for the upper and lower right quadrants and thanked me profusely for "doing exactly what we discussed." As I walked her out towards the exit, she appeared to almost float out our front door while her daughter looked on in amazement.

CASE #9

This case was one that I felt was incomplete. My patient had definitely been helped by his one NLP session, but he could have used two additional sessions to get the results he said he wanted. However, he was pleased with his results and was not willing to schedule any more sessions.

JC came to me with the chief concern of needing a root canal but unable to complete the treatment when he was at the Endodontist's office. He said that the rubber dam used for protection during the procedure was placed in his mouth and he "immediately became anxious, felt closed in, couldn't breathe and had to stop the treatment and get out of the office." He seemed extremely uncomfortable talking one on one with me and when I gently asked about it he told me, "I never thought I would need help for something like this. I can control my life and do anything I want to do, and this annoys me and makes me feel ridiculous. I just want to be able to get my root canal finished."

Even with his resistance and difficulty accepting his issue, I was able to uncover valuable information that would allow me to help him. I learned that he realized that his tolerance in a dental chair had become less over time. His sleep apnea would kick in when he was laid back in a dental chair and he could not breathe once the rubber dam was placed. He said, "I just panic, fearing that I can't breathe."

During our session together, he allowed me to guide him in a visualization using the movie theatre process, taking him back to his last appointment. I asked him to remember what it was like and to notice as much as he could from a safer "looking back" perspective. I helped him to "reframe" the incident (look at it a different way), by offering the suggestion that even though the rubber dam was used for his protection, his "natural knowing" and "unconscious" was trying to protect him, which is a very good thing. I asked him to re-visualize the same situation and consider what could be added or changed to help him breathe better, comfort him and allow him to get the procedure accomplished.

JC was able to come up with an action plan that he felt he could live with and decided that was enough for the session and he wanted it ended. He refused any other tools, anchors, suggestions or NLP sessions.

Before ending his session, I calibrated that he visually appeared less anxious talking about returning to the Endodontist's office and his body language was consistent with what he was saying. His newfound confidence and determination showed in his stature and he thanked me and left.

Later that day he called my office to tell me that he had called the endodontist and scheduled an appointment. We did not hear from JC until after this root canal was completed. He came back to my office to have the post and core and crown done.

He related to me that he was glad he got through his root canal treatment and was able to withstand the rubber dam for a short period of time. He confirmed that the work we had done together had helped him accomplish it.

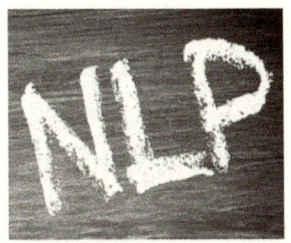

CASE #10

BB arrived saying, "I am terrified of having any dental work at all done, I want to be in control at all times and I'm really afraid you're going to put me under." She said she wanted to know everything I was going to do.

I stopped my questioning and shared with her the process of my NLP and that there is "no going under," just an opportunity to discover where her anxieties come from if she wants to know. I also told her that I could help her to add "tools and resources" to help her better deal with those anxieties or completely eliminate them if that was what she wanted.

As I listened to her, she talked about "the long creepy hallway leading to the dentist's office and hearing the screeching of the drill and feeling trapped in the reception area." She said, "I felt like there was no turning back and I couldn't refuse treatment. I lost my voice completely."

She said she clearly remembers the male dentist gave her an injection and she felt like she was choking. The dentist took out two teeth and her mouth was full of blood and she was panicking. Then she remembered "shutting down" and unable to say much and leaving the office never to return again.

BB told me, "That experience floods my mind whenever I think of going to a dentist, so I have not returned for many years."

When I asked her what her goal was working with me she replied, "What I want is to seek dental care feeling calm, peaceful and unafraid and in control." I talked with her about the process of visualization and that before we began, we needed to install some positive anchors to help her and protect her from the trauma she remembered experiencing. She agreed and we began her NLP appointment.

I had her relax in her chair and close her eyes, as I guided her to her safe place. Then, I added in the positive resources she said she wanted and anchored them on her left wrist. I tested the resource anchor and when it was firmly established, I asked her to imagine being in a movie theater and proceeded to guide her through a visualization of her past experience reinforcing that she was now in a very safe place, far, far away from the action she was watching.

She was very resistant at first trying to control her images but eventually she said she could feel and trust her "safe" anchor and allowed the visualization to flow naturally. I calibrated her arms and legs resting completely against her chair, watched her face loosen up and noticed a turning up of both corners of her lips. She then said: "I know what I need now. Somehow the past doesn't seem as gruesome and horrific as it used to."

I calibrated that her body was in alignment with what she had just said and I tested the anchor, confirmed it was working well and then future paced her. When I was done, her lips broke into a huge grin; she gave a slight laugh and said out loud; "I am feeling so much better now."

Her action plan for her dental appointments included: being the first patient of the day, being seated right away and not left waiting in the reception area, having the dentist or assistant stay in the room with her at all times and getting as much done at each appointment as possible. She wanted to know what was going on at all times and to be in control and able to stop if needed. As she outlined her needs she was holding tightly onto her resource anchor as I had directed and she acted much more relaxed and confident.

We scheduled a treatment appointment two weeks later and when she returned she did quite well. At the completion of her dental appointment she sat up, looked directly at me and said, "That's absolutely amazing. I thought back to the past for a minute and it didn't affect me or make me anxious at all. Thank you so much."

HAVE NO FEAR OF THE DENTAL CHAIR!

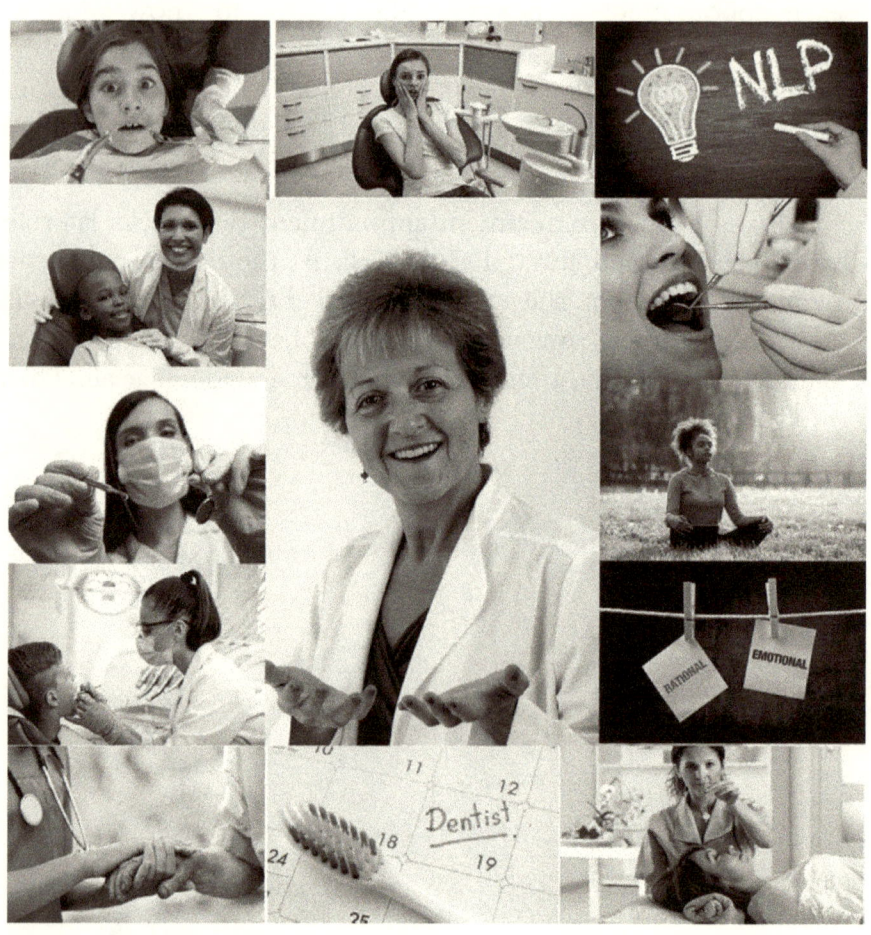

CASE #11

This case was probably one of the most amazing stories I have witnessed so far of a complete 180 degree turn around from dental phobia to a calm and relaxed state.

JM arrived to my office saying: "I have a hole in my tooth and it hurts." I noticed that he was slightly pale and appeared very stiff. When I brought him into the operatory, he stood standing and would not take a seat in the operatory chair. I reviewed his medical and dental history, as I did with all my patients planning on having dental treatment, and asked his permission to "take a brief look inside his mouth." He reluctantly agreed and then sat half way in the dental chair all the while keeping his right foot firmly planted on the floor. I asked him to lean back and try to relax in the chair while I did my brief exam.

As I did so, I could see sweat beading up on his forehead and his body slightly shaking. I completed my exam quickly and as soon as I stopped looking in his mouth, he immediately sat upright, put both of his feet on the floor, gripped the arm rest and stared directly ahead through the picture window.

I asked him some questions about his dental history and his concerns and I saw sweat dripping from his face onto his shirt. I could see that he was sweating profusely all over, slightly shaking and barely breathing. I shared with him my personal history of dental anxiety and what happened to change that for me. I added in some NLP pre-suppositions to be used for future reference, in order to help him relax and expect a painless appointment. It was also to offer him positive reframing and resources that could help him later on.

I reviewed the X-ray that was taken and saw that there was a deep cavity into the pulp (the nerve inside of the tooth) and told him that he had two choices. He could save the tooth with a root canal (removal of the nerve and infection), a post and core (to rebuild the inside of the tooth) and a crown (restoring the outside of the tooth) or he could have an extraction (removal of the infected tooth). I then listed all the anxiety reducing techniques I offered. The list seemed to help his anxiety a bit but he was still unable to look at me for more than a second at a time and seemed speechless.

When he could finally speak, he told me that he wanted to save his tooth and thought that he needed an NLP-AMC session or two before he could ever let me start any dental treatment. I sent him home with pamphlets on the various treatments he would need and also gave him my personal phone number in case he needed to talk to me personally. JM made an appointment to return three days later for his NLP session.

When he returned three days later, I began the session by asking him what he wanted. All he could do was look away in the distance and say, "I just want to be able to get this tooth fixed without this panic I'm feeling." He said that he did not know why he was so terrified since he could not remember any specific past dental trauma. However, from my experience, I was sure that he had to have had at least one if not many that were blocked in his unconscious memory.

I asked him if he could put his desires in positive terms because NLP works by using positive directives and not negative commands. (Research has shown that our brains hear commands of what we want rather than what we do not want.) After what seemed like a very long time, JM said, "I want to be relaxed at the dental office."

I spent quite some time working with him to identify positive resources he could draw on. Once he determined what positive resources he wanted I anchored them on his right arm, where it would be easily accessible for both of us to reach. Then, I held onto his resource-safety anchor as I slowly guided him through a "Double Disassociation Phobia Removal Process." I asked him to visualize whatever traumatic dental image he kept seeing in his mind, and watch it playing on a very, far away screen lined with double-thick Plexiglas for his protection. I had him run his movie over and over many times, including backwards, forwards and in small sections until I calibrated a definite change in his state.

In addition to the kinesthetic anchor on his right arm, I decided to add auditory and visual anchors that could be used later on during his dental treatment. I felt that he needed these additional positive resources in order for me to help him get past whatever was blocking him.

I also decided to install a second physical-safety anchor in a more accessible location (his right palm) for him to use when he needed it. When I tested it, JM told me it was in the perfect spot and felt quite powerful to him. Once we were both confident that it worked exactly the way he desired, I future paced it for him. He told me that he believed he was as ready as he would ever be and asked if we could start his root canal that day.

So, I led JM to a dental operatory, started the nitrous oxide and began my Milton Model, hypnotic languaging. When I calibrated a slight relaxation and felt the dose of nitrous was good for him, I placed the topical anesthetic in his mouth. I told him what I was doing and anesthetized his tooth.

As I performed the root canal treatment, I triggered the anchor on his right arm and saw his anxiety decreasing. When the root canal treatment was completed, I lowered the percentage of the nitrous oxide and placed him on only oxygen to flush out his system and to allow him to get back to normal. By the end of the appointment, I noticed that he was no longer sweating and his body seemed more relaxed. I added in some pre-suppositions for his next appointment and some more future pacing.

When we were done, I sat him up and JM looked directly into my eyes for the first time, smiled and said, "That was great! I didn't feel any pain at all." JM then asked me if he could schedule his next appointment soon. We scheduled the post and crown appointment two weeks later.

When JM came into the office, two weeks later, he greeted my receptionist with a big smile, appeared visibly relaxed and was seated in an operatory. We began to place the nitrous mask on his nose and he stated, "I feel relaxed. I don't need the nitrous today." We were quite surprised but very pleased for him. I placed the topical anesthetic, anesthetized his tooth and performed the post and crown treatment.

At subsequent appointments, I did his other treatment needs and he continued to remain relaxed and comfortable at all of them needing only the local anesthetic.

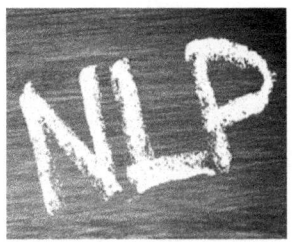

CASE #12

MB arrived with her chief concern being, "I have a broken tooth, it's been hurting on and off for four weeks and increasing in pain the last few days." He said to me, "I hate the drill noise and if I could have dental work without it, I think I might be able to get through it." He said he had tried headphones, but could still hear the noise and said, "It makes me crazy." He wanted to try NLP and see if that could help him better deal with the noises.

After getting to know him better by asking leading questions and asking about his desired outcome and what triggers and resources he had, I decided to "install" an auditory anchor of "hearing his children's voices and laughter" in addition to a kinesthetic anchor of "feeling spiritual feelings I get whenever I work at the soup kitchen", whenever he heard a dental drill. When I tested them, he told me: "That's amazing, I feel wonderful." He said he was ready and requested an appointment for the following day. I discussed his dental needs and suggested he use the nitrous oxide as an adjunct and he willingly agreed.

When he came in the next day, I placed him on nitrous oxide, anesthetized his tooth and surgically removed his severely fractured tooth using my drill. When the procedure was done, he remarked, "I can't believe that worked so well. I could hear a drill being used, but then it changed into my kids laughing and my helping out at my soup kitchen. It was great."

When he returned a few weeks later to see the hygienist, he told her, "No gas today, I will be fine." And he was!

CASE #13

GP arrived to my office saying, "I am terrified of dentists and I always pass out or get sick and not always in that order." GP proceeded to tell us that she was leaving in one month as a guide for a diving expedition out of the country and needed her teeth cleaned and fixed before she went. She said, "It's been a few years since I have seen a dentist, but one of my teeth hurt and it has to get fixed before I dive." I noticed that she was clenching the arm of the dental chair, was leaning away from me as she spoke, her face was pale while her eyes were gazing right through me and she kept her feet on the floor the entire time.

She seemed resistant to my suggestion to return for a private NLP session, so I took the opportunity to do as much NLP during the examination and interview process as I could. We spent enough time together for me to gain good rapport and find out enough about her to help install some auditory and visual anchors with her permission. The visual anchor that she chose as her "relaxing scene" was "tagging sharks," a very different scenario than I would have imagined. I learned a lot from her that day about my taking "second position" (objective perspective) and to always come from my patient's "map of the world," (viewpoint or paradigm), and not my own.

I suggested that when she returned for a treatment appointment we would use these anchors along with the nitrous oxide. She considered this for a moment, consented and requested an appointment for the next day.

The following day, I placed her on nitrous oxide and used Milton Modeling and NLP languaging along with her anchors. Her treatment went very smoothly and at the end, she smiled and said, "I can't believe I actually got through it!"

Meanwhile unbeknownst to me, her husband had shown up at the office during her appointment asking my receptionist what hospital his wife was at so that he could pick her up. He explained to my receptionist that every dental appointment GP had ever had, had caused her to faint or get so ill that she ended up at the hospital. When he was told that she was doing well he could not believe it. As I brought her out of the operatory she was smiling and we both went to meet him in the reception area. I noticed that he was staring at us and heard him saying out loud: "That's just amazing."

Then, GP said to him, "Dr. Cushing is incredible. I have never been able to get through a dental appointment before today." He came over to us, hugged his wife and then shook my hand. He looked quite shocked, but also very relieved.

GP returned to my office many times for her recall (cleaning and examination) and treatment appointments and continued to do quite well.

CASE #14

Dealing with anxious patients that become angry and hostile are a concern for most dentists. NLP can also be used to help manage these people better.

GB arrived to my office acting very angry and belligerent. When she approached the front desk, she verbally attacked my receptionist and was very rude to my dental assistant. When I heard what was going on, I looked out from my operatory and I calibrated her tense body, piercing eyes, loud voice coming out in guttural tones, aggressive stance and heard her making demands.

My well-trained dental assistant treated GB with extreme kindness and asked how she could help her. The only thing GB would say was that, "My mouth hurts and I want it taken care of now." This was not the first time this particularly anxious patient had felt free enough to dump her anger and hostility onto my staff and me. She had an angry demeanor, but it became unbearable when she was in pain.

I fully understood her concerns and I sympathized with her frustration and empathized with her pain. However, I knew that I could not allow this abusive behavior anymore. Her behavior had begun to upset all of us enough that it affected how we viewed our day; how we were able to treat her and left all of us emotionally drained once she left.

Let me mention here that after becoming a Master Practitioner of NLP, I decided to use my skills for most of my daily communication with everyone I came into contact with. I would review in my mind prior conversations I had had with challenging and difficult people and consider what I could have said or done differently to have influenced the outcomes into a more positive result. So, that's exactly what I decided to do when I heard GB in my office that day.

I realized that I cared about this patient and what must be underlying all her animosity and intimidating behavior. I wondered if the process of pacing and leading could help with my next communication with her especially if I were to be completely honest and direct. I was fully aware that only a small fraction of our communication with others is verbal and if my body language and tone of my words didn't reflect the rest of my communicating, it would only make things worse.

So, I slowly walked into the operatory, where my assistant had seated her, I said hello to GB and sat down in my chair. I slid over next to her and slightly in front of her at the same level. I could actually feel the negative energy of fierce aggression and hostility coming out of her. I offered a pleasant greeting and asked how I could help her. GB proceeded to tell me that she wasn't feeling well, her tooth and gums hurt, the other doctor she had seen had made it worse and then said: "You better take care of it now". [Note - She had actually improperly re-cemented her own temporary crown with super glue and caused her own side effects, but was unwilling to accept her accountability and resultant circumstances.]

I followed her lead by sitting fully erect in my chair and restated loudly and firmly what GB had said to me. I said, "I hear what you are saying and it sounds like you aren't feeling well and your tooth and gums hurt. I am sorry that you are uncomfortable and I am here to clear things up."

GB aggressively said, "Well just do it then, just take care of it and get it done." I stopped and took a deep breath, sat her chair up a bit more forward and said firmly and in a voice matching her, "GB, I truly care about you. My patients are my friends and mean a lot to me and in this practice I only treat my friends. You and I have been together for a while now and I would like to continue that. I have considered you a friend, however your aggressive behavior is getting worse and I cannot allow it any longer. I understand that you are frustrated, upset, and in pain, but taking it out on us is not acceptable. We want to do all we can to help you. You are the one that re-cemented your temporary with superglue and there are side effects and consequences to that. I need you to be patient and allow us to help you."

GB jumped in and yelled at me: "So you are blaming me, the patient. That's not the way to treat a patient!" I responded to her by saying, "I am not blaming anyone. However, the fact is that when you decided to use super glue to re-cement your temporary there were consequences that you are now experiencing. I will do all I can to correct it, get you out of pain and restore your tooth to comfort and health, but you must be patient, treat us with kindness and respect, just as we treat you."

GB then said, "I can't believe you said that to me. You need to learn communication skills and how to talk to your patients. Just leave me alone." I, then, restated in a slightly softer tone that I cared about her and that I could only help her if she let me. I reminded her that she has to trust me and understand how my staff and I feel when she is rude and directs her anger at us. I said, "If you do not want me to treat you, it is just fine. You can leave whenever you want. However, if you want your dental problems treated here, then, I need to tell you what we expect from you."

[Let me note here that the entire time we were talking, I was mirroring her body language and her voice, pacing and leading trying to be in rapport.]

After a few minutes of silence had passed, GB said, "Just go ahead, it's fine." I calibrated that she was a bit less aggressive in her body tenseness and she had lain back in the chair in a more open, "vulnerable" position.

So I said, "GB, let me gently lay you back, do my exam and evaluate exactly what I can do to help you." She allowed me to do so and after the examination was completed, I sat her back up. I explained what needed to be done, the time it would take and what results she could expect.

Surprisingly, she said, "I'm sorry if I was rude to you and your staff, it's just that I have been feeling so terrible and afraid what was going on. I didn't realize it was as bad as you said it was."

I responded, "I'm sure that it wasn't your intention, but it is how it came out. We all just want to be able to take care of your dental needs and we can only do that if there is honesty and mutual respect. I accept your apology."

When GB left my operatory, she was in a much different state than I had ever seen her in. She walked over to the front desk and apologized to my receptionist for being rude saying she would be careful in the future. Then, she sought out my dental assistant and did the same.

GB returned many times after that appointment and never treated any one of us rudely or with hostility again. I even noticed that when she came in experiencing other dental issues and began to become agitated and aggressive, she would back off and restate her situation in a more receptive tone. It became a pleasure to treat her and very rewarding for all of us.

CASE #15

FP was a patient assigned to me when I worked as an associate dentist after selling my first dental practice in Boise, Idaho. The owner dentist told me he had a "highly phobic" female patient that he had designated as "prophy only" (a prophy is a dental cleaning) because she was willing to schedule her cleaning appointments with his hygienist, but that was all. The dentist had noted that the longer the time interval between her operative appointments (fillings, crowns), the more her phobia increased. He said that he had completed all her dental work quite a few years ago, but recently she had presented to his office with severe pain and needed a root canal.

He told me that the root canal had gone well from his viewpoint, but she had not returned since to have the necessary post and crown done. He had called her to schedule an appointment, but she refused. He knew of her dental fear, but thought she might be mildly depressed and suggested she seek treatment with a therapist.

I asked the receptionist to schedule her next prophy appointment when I was in the office, so I could meet her and perform her six month dental exam. When FP came in I was able to develop rapport immediately and she shared with me that when her tooth hurt and she had the root canal, she was so afraid that even though she knew she was numb, that she had still felt pain and it "freaked her out." She said, "Now just the thought of feeling pain makes me cry and I cry at all my dental appointments, even the cleanings." She told me that she had tried the nitrous oxide once and really loved it, but didn't think it would be enough, because she can't even schedule the appointment to come in.

I learned that she started to obsess about her dental appointment weeks ahead of time and would think to herself, "What if I feel pain?, What if something happens during my appointment, What if the anesthetic isn't strong enough or I lose the numbness too quickly?" She said, "My fear of the *unknown* looms largely in my mind and actually creates a sense of pain when I sit in the chair."

As I sat next to her, I could tell that she was comfortable with me and I began to ask more probing questions, all the while using my NLP and hypnotic languaging. She said that all her childhood dental experiences were very traumatic. She said, "My mother would have to drag me hysterical and crying, while I shook uncontrollably." She had developed anxiety of all pain in general as a result of being picked on and bullied by kids when she was a child.

She remembered a particularly horrible incident where she went to the dentist and was "strapped down while they put a gas mask on my nose and I bawled and screamed while they pulled my tooth. Since then, I go to an oral surgeon and get Valium to get infected teeth taken out."

I explained to her how NLP counseling worked and asked if she wanted to try a session that day. She told me it sounded interesting and she felt she could trust me and agreed.

I considered all the possible processes that might work for her and chose the "Phobic Removal process" and the "Memory

Release-Reframe with Changing Personal History process (changing a negative memory into a positive memory). First, I assessed and verified her ecology, making sure she was ready for change and would not be harmed in any way. I calibrated that all her body language and external signs were congruent and then I made sure that she was clear about what she wanted. She told me she really wanted to get rid of her phobia, because her teeth were very important to her and she was ready. She added that her mother had lost all of her teeth from lack of dental care and developing gum disease and FP was determined to do all she could to avoid the same thing for herself.

I used one of my NLP-Hypnotic languaging patterns and watched as her body began relaxing and sloping comfortably in her chair. I calibrated minimal fidgeting as she allowed herself to get more and more settled. Her hands that were usually very expressive and moved about continuously were now lying quietly on her lap.

I asked her to imagine something that gave her strength and safety and with her permission added a resource-safety anchor on her right wrist. This would help her stay balanced and safe when I elicited the past trauma from her. I tested the anchor and decided it needed more power and continued to work with her until she added in more resources that gave both of us the confidence to proceed.

I had her access the past dental experience that kept coming to her mind filling her with fear and blocking out her resolve to go to the dentist. Next, I asked her to run the memory backwards, forwards and to jumble it up as much as she could. As she did so, I continued to hold onto her right wrist anchor allowing it to counterbalance the memory and defuse the intensity of it. When I noted that she was not reacting and was maintaining her calm, I asked her to consider what she would have liked to have had happen and who she wished had been there offering safety and support. This was a much longer process. As I guided FP through this, I worked with her as she added in the various tools and attributes needed as well as the outside support she wanted until she had created her "ideal scenario."

I told her to run a movie of that "ideal scenario" a few times from beginning to end, seeing, hearing and feeling all she could get from it, and when what she envisioned felt absolutely "perfect" to her to give me a sign that she was done. After a few minutes, FP nodded her head and I installed a second anchor on her right forearm while simultaneously triggering her "safety" resource anchor on her right wrist. When she was prepared to come out of this "trance state," I rechecked her ecology again. Calibrating that everything was good, I future paced with her while I combined both of her anchors into one, whereby both strengthening and having only one powerful anchor for her to use. She slowly opened her eyes and when she spoke she looked and sounded quite different from the woman who had originally asked me for help.

She told me she actually felt different and was anxious to start dental treatment with me. We scheduled an appointment the following Monday and I gave her an assignment to practice using her resource anchor when she felt it could be useful. She agreed and asked if she could give me a hug, which I gratefully accepted.

FP came to her appointment on Monday looking poised and prepared to get her treatment done. When I greeted her she told me she had practiced using her anchor at home and at work and was amazed that it helped her keep her composure and stay calm and stand up for herself, when normally she would have felt worried and intimidated. She said that she was anxious to get today's appointment under her belt to prove that her dental phobia was a thing of the past.

I offered her a music CD with headphones that she accepted and we began. She did extremely well with the anesthetic and appeared comfortable throughout the drilling portion. I stopped a few times to check in with her and she assured me that she was doing well. She seemed to have found serenity and a newfound confidence. I noticed that she triggered her anchor a few times during the procedure, but as we neared the end of her treatment she had her hands resting fully on her lap and was no longer touching her anchor.

The appointment went extremely well and at the end she removed her headphones and gave me a huge smile and said, "That was incredible! I had no panic inside and I totally trusted you and was able to relax into the music. Thank you so much. I will definitely be coming regularly from now on." Which she did.

HAVE NO FEAR OF THE DENTAL CHAIR!

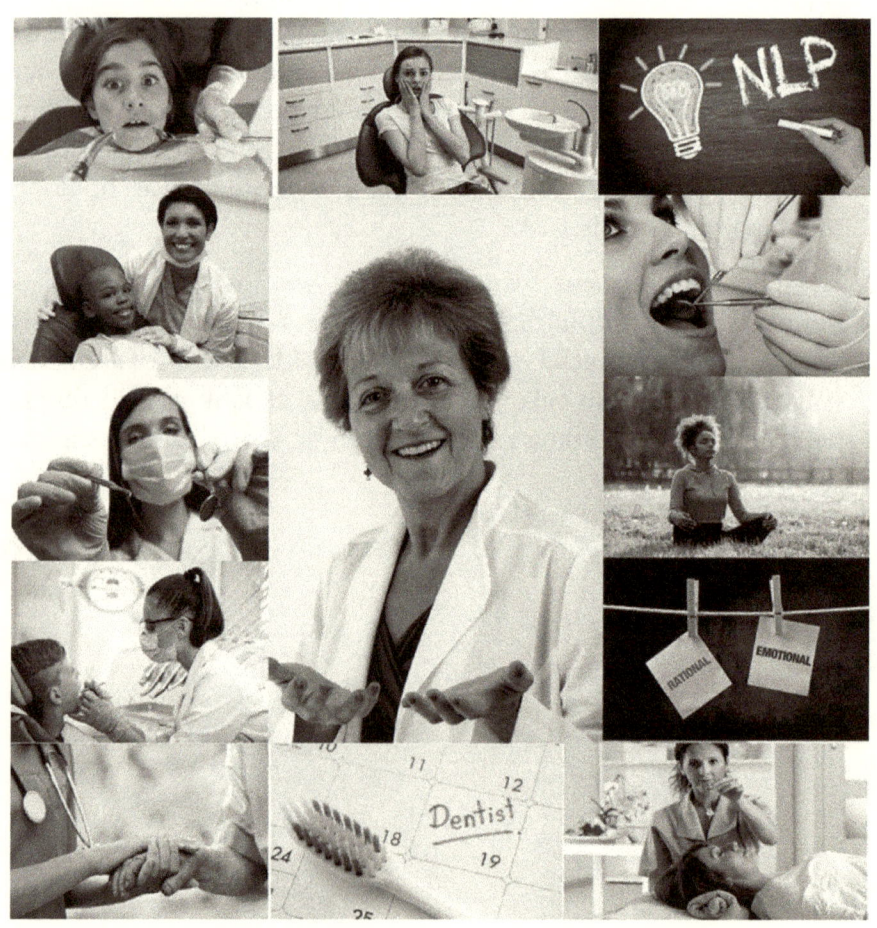

CASE #16

This case was probably my funniest one. My friend, StD came to me telling me he wanted to repair some old fractured fillings, but had some anxiety and kept putting it off. He said that he had no traumatic past experiences but knew that he had just gotten more anxious as he got older. He firmly stated that he did not want to have any NLP sessions.

After reviewing his health history and dental history, I did not find any specific anxiety or fear for us to work on. I felt that using the nitrous oxide alone might be just the added ingredient to make him comfortable. When I suggested it to him, he told me he had never used it before, but had heard from others it was helpful and decided to try it. He requested we start his dental treatment that day. So, we took a full series of X-rays, performed a comprehensive examination and then I reviewed my findings with him. I suggested a treatment plan and what we should begin with. He consented and I placed him on the nitrous oxide starting at 30% and then raising it to 40% at which time he said: "This stuff is good, you can start anytime."

So, I placed the topical anesthetic in his mouth and anesthetized the area I would be treating. I calibrated that he was doing really well and the procedure went quite quickly. After I completed my work and removed his nose mask, he was grinning from ear to ear, looking like the "cat that had swallowed the canary." I sat him up and asked what he thought about the treatment and specifically about using the nitrous. His answer surprised me, when he said, "Well, It was a spiritual experience. I was transported back in time to my hippy days when I experimented with drugs and I saw God. It was amazing."

CASE #17

DF was one of my simpler cases. She came to her NLP-AMC session saying: "I haven't been to a dentist for over 5 years, I've been too afraid. My front teeth are loose and I need them out so I can get a denture, but I can't make an appointment, I get too upset." She sat straight up in the chair fidgeting and appearing very afraid. She said, "Anytime I think back to past dental appointments, I get agitated and can't do anything."

I calibrated her closely as I asked about her medical history, her dental history, her family, her job and her desires. With this information, I was able to get her strategy process. I determined that it would be best to get her a positive, resourceful state with anchors before we talked any more about her past.

When I asked DF what she was looking for, she responded with the following statement: "When I go to the dentist, I want to feel like I do when I think of my two and a half year old daughter." She shared with me that after many difficult years of trying to conceive a child and then many more frustrating years of trying to adopt a child, she was finally able to find an adoption agency and adopt her daughter. She said, "I absolutely adore my daughter and feel such incredible joy and complete success about the whole thing."

Using this information as the basis, I helped install this resource as an anchor for her to use whenever it was appropriate. I tested it and then future paced her being sure to have her imagine what it would be like when she had her teeth removed and when she went for all her future appointments. I calibrated that her anchor was powerful and readily available to her. When she left my consult room she looked content, uplifted and ready to make an appointment with the oral surgeon for that Friday.

When I called her Saturday post operatively, she stated, "I got it done. I had my tops pulled. You would have been so proud of me." She returned in two weeks for the denture process and told me that she trusted me and was totally comfortable getting work done now that she had her resource anchor for support.

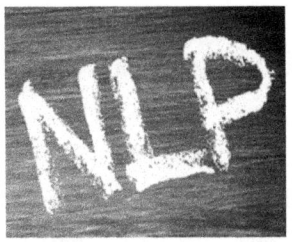

CASE #18

BH is one of my favorite and most memorable patients.

BH was a four year old boy who came to me because he had been turned away by two general dentists and a Pedodontist, (a dental specialist dealing with children). His mother had been told that he would have to be treated in a hospital setting using IV sedation (General Anesthesia). She told me that she had minimal funds and did not want her son treated with General Anesthesia.

She said that at the dental appointments, BH was anxious and unable to sit in a dental chair. All the dentists had told her that he was too apprehensive to treat in a dental office and that he was uncooperative. She said that one dentist even yelled at him and made him cry, which increased his anxiety.

BH's mom, a dental phobic herself, told me very firmly that she did not want her little boy getting his dental care in a hospital. Then she said: "I have been referred to you by the Pedodontist-specialist as a last resort."

I sat down next to BH and immediately noticed his apprehension and anxiety. His eyes had been following me while I spoke to his mother and continued to stare directly at me. I immediately noticed how fragile he appeared and how he seemed to really want to cooperate.

I introduced myself as Dr. C and began to ask him questions so I could get to know him. He was a delightful child and easy to get into rapport with. I told him my own stories of being afraid of the dentist and how it all changed for me.

After some time, I felt he could handle more. So, I asked if I could do an examination and he agreed. I led him to a treatment room and asked permission to look at his teeth and he slowly opened his mouth. I hinted that it might tickle him and that he could stop me at any time by raising his left hand. The entire time I encouraged him and told him just how brave he was. I added in pre-suppositions and verbal anchors for future positive behavior and my expectations.

I learned that he had a rabbit that he loved very much, had some dogs and loved stories.

[Note - I assumed his rabbit was real since he spoke of it as if it were. However later on I found out it was actually a stuffed rabbit! This became a very important lesson for me when treating children. He was much more cooperative than I had expected and I was sure that we could work together.]

The next few days I wrote a special metaphor for him, telling the story about Hector, the rabbit (my personal pet at the time), who had gotten a thorn in his paw and was afraid to see the doctor. However, since Hector trusted me so much and knew I would NEVER do anything to hurt him if possible (presupposition using hypnotic languaging added throughout), he let me bring him to see "DocSee" (Dr. C is what I have children call me). I also added in the presupposition that Hector could raise his left paw ANYTIME he got scared or needed to take a break. I made sure to add that he must leave his right arm on the arm rest so DocSee could easily reach him to take care of him.

I ended the story with how Hector was so surprised how easy it was, how little it really hurt, how much better he felt when DocSee was done, how proud he was of himself and how much he liked DocSee for taking such good care of him.

BH returned to my office the following Tuesday. I sat with him in my consult room and proceeded to share the story of Hector, the rabbit. As I told the story, BH appeared mesmerized and quickly got into a trance. I calibrated just how involved he was throughout and made mental notes of specific reactions and ways I could use parts of the story at a later time.

At the end of the story, I asked if he would like to visit all of our special rooms where Dr. C takes care of our patients. He seemed relaxed, yet excited to go. My assistant and I took him on a brief tour and then found a "special chair" just for him. He sat in the chair and I showed him the "space mask" (nitrous oxide mask). I explained how it worked and how much fun he could have if he wanted to.

Then, I reviewed with both he and his mother what the next visit would be like and asked him if he would come back and visit us again "real soon". He seemed quite ready and we made an appointment.

BH and his mom returned that Friday. I took his hand and led him alone to his "special chair", placed the nitrous mask on his nose letting him adjust it as he needed to and telling him that he could ask a question or stop us at any time he needed to by just raising his left hand.

I sat next to him and reminded him about his rabbit and about Hector and how DocSee had helped Hector. As I started the nitrous I began using "Milton Modeling" hypnotic language and BH abruptly raised his left hand (signaling us to stop) and I stopped and asked what he needed. BH seemed to be smiling but said nothing, just lowered his hand. He was simply "testing" us. After two more of these "tests," to determine if he could trust us, especially me, I was able to trance him using sections of the metaphor I'd written for him. I placed the topical in his mouth, anesthetized him and when he was numb I drilled and filled the teeth we had planned on doing that day.

When we were done, I turned off the nitrous and flushed his system using only oxygen and then I sat him up. I told him how terrific he did, how both Hector and DocSee would be so proud of him and how we would like to see him back again real soon.

He looked directly at me, smiled and said he'd like to come back. I then took his hand and together we went to meet his mother in the reception room. When she saw us she looked shocked to see her little boy smiling and holding my hand. I reviewed what we had done, how well he did and what was left to complete. I told BH to be very careful not to bite his cheek or tongue and only eat after the numbness was gone.

I asked BH if I could have a hug and he gave me a huge hug that brought tears to my eyes (and still does this many years later). We brought out a treasure chest box and while he chose a prize, his mother scheduled another appointment.

On subsequent appointments, BH did just as well. He continued to return for his six months Recare (cleaning and examination) appointments.

[Note- At one of BH's first Recare appointments, he and I were chatting and I found out that his rabbit was not a real one. Actually it was a stuffed animal that he had gotten when he was very young and was his favorite. I asked if he wanted a real rabbit one day and he said, yes.]

Interestingly enough, I had just had two experiences with my rabbit, Hector, where I had gotten some of his fur in my eyes and had a severe allergic reaction from the dander and ended up at the Emergency Room (ER). At the ER they told me it would get worse with each exposure and I should either be very careful around Hector or find another home for him. I was very reluctant to do so, because I loved Hector, but was worried about what could happen if I did get exposed again.

So, I met with BH's mother and asked how she felt about getting her son a real rabbit. She said that they owned a big farm and had all kinds of animals but no rabbit and if BH would take care of it, she would welcome the idea. We both knew how much BH had wanted a rabbit and just what Hector and DocSee had done for her son.

Then, that weekend, she and BH came to my house and met Hector and it was "love at first sight." BH stood at the side of the cage and Hector sniffed his fingers while they played and his mother said, "Okay, you can have him." I was so pleased that my Hector now had a new person that would love him and care for him and it felt so right that my story was now completed.

HAVE NO FEAR OF THE DENTAL CHAIR!

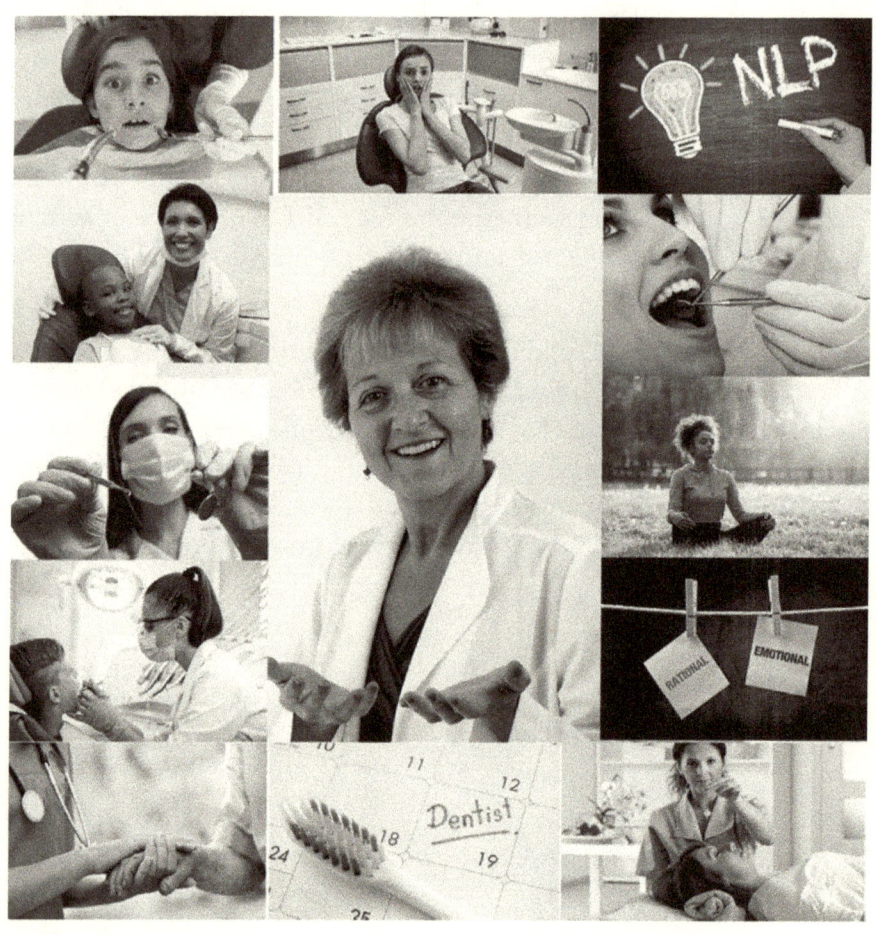

CASE #19

This is another very interesting case and one that not only tells a story of fear, but also teaches us that people can be pre-judged and misdiagnosed by dentists. Doing so can create phobias and doubts about what we as patients feel we know.

In this case BC had absolutely no dental anxiety or fear until it was created by a dental scenario that made her question her own sanity. This patient was made to feel like her symptoms were something other than she believed them to be and was negated by the "dental professionals."

BC came to see me for a consult and second opinion, saying she was never afraid of a dentist until her recent experiences scared her and made her distrustful and afraid. She said that she went to a Community Health Clinic saying she had intense pain on her left side, starting in her lower left tooth and radiating all the way to her left jaw. She was told by the treating dental student extern that she had "TMJ" and would need a mouth guard to help relieve her TMJ (Temporomandibular Joint) pain. The student told her she had a cavity in her lower right molar that had to be treated before she could have her mouth guard made, so it would fit correctly. She agreed and he began treatment.

She said she was surprised that there was no supervising dentist around, but felt uncomfortable saying anything so she didn't. She then related the following story to me: "The student placed the topical anesthetic on the top of my teeth and not on my gum like I was sure he was supposed to. Then he gave me the shot that lasted five minutes and was absolutely the most painful shot I had ever had. He hit my lip and I felt this incredible jolt of electric pain. I was in pain and I started to tell him, but he rather abruptly told me not to talk so he could get his work done. He drilled my tooth for an hour and when his friend came in and asked why he was still drilling he told him: "I have to make sure all the decay is gone, I'm drilling more to be sure". Meanwhile, an instructor never came in to check on him and I thought that was odd. When he was filling my tooth, he banged it so hard that it shook my face and when he kept it up I started to have terrible pain in my entire face. Then the left side of my face began to throb and I could feel my left TMJ begin to ache. I am still in a lot of pain in both my jaws since that appointment. I finally left the clinic and after the anesthetic wore off I was in a lot of pain. When I called the clinic, I was told to take Ibuprofen and it would go away soon.

The pain did not go away and I have been to the Emergency Room three times since then and all they would do was give me OxyContin that made me sick and gave me hallucinations. I finally was offered an appointment and able to see a "real dentist" at the clinic who told me I had "irreversible pulpitis" on my lower right molar with the new silver filling and I needed a root canal and crown. I was upset, because I never had any pain before I went there and now my tooth won't stop hurting, my entire face and jaw hurts and I cannot fully close my mouth, especially on the lower left side. I have never had TMJ problems and if I have them it's from all the banging he did on my tooth when he filled it. And I am still feeling pain on my lower left side. I am so afraid of what might be wrong and afraid to trust anyone."

In this case I used my NLP techniques of asking many questions all the while listening, back tracking, and pacing and leading in order to get the complete story and develop rapport and trust. Due to this patient's anxiety and coming in for only a "consultation", we decided to keep her appointment brief and to determine if indeed she needed a root canal and crown on the tooth in question. She did allow me to take one new radiograph of the lower right molar and do a limited examination of that area.

As I listened to her symptoms, I asked her if she could close her mouth evenly or if she felt one side of her mouth was higher than the other side. Interestingly enough, she looked at me intensely and said, "I cannot close my mouth on the left side. Since I had the filling done by the student dentist, my teeth only touch on my right side." I took out some marking paper and checked her bite and noted she was hitting only on her new silver filling. With her permission, I adjusted and recontoured the filling after verifying it with the indicating paper. After a couple of adjustments, she sat up straight in the chair and smiled and said, "Wow…that feels so much better. Now I can finally close on my left side."

Since I wanted to allow a little time for her tooth to heal and to determine if her pain was reversible or irreversible nerve pain, I decided to have her return the following week for a comprehensive examination and determine if there was any change in her pain on the right side. When there is a "high spot" on a tooth after a filling or crown has been done, the stresses from eating can cause pain and inflammation underneath the tooth, feeling like a blister. You can think of it as having "a rock in your shoe" that rubs all day and eventually causes pain when you walk. I told her to try eating normally on both sides and notice if the pain on the right side was decreasing or not. She thanked me for seeing her, said she felt she could trust me, and thanked me for finding a high spot and giving her time to see if a root canal was needed.

BC returned the next week complaining that she was experiencing extreme pain on the left back molar and it did not feel like TMJ. She allowed us to take a radiograph of the offending tooth and another of the lower right tooth. Low and behold, when I reviewed the new radiograph, there was a huge abscess underneath her lower left back molar. Her instinct and sense of pain was indeed on target. I showed it to her on our digital screen, prescribed her antibiotics and referred her to the Endodontist, (a specialist that does root canals) to have a root canal done. The radiograph showed no abscess on the lower right molar at that time and she said she had no pain or discomfort at all from the lower right tooth or from her TMJ.

As I pondered what BC had gone through at the clinic, I kept thinking that she had allowed the student dentist to "hurt her" in order to be a good patient, all the while trusting that he would fix her problem. She had fought her gut instinct "to get away from the clinic" believing "a dental student and a real dentist should know more than she did." She said she felt there was definitely something wrong on her lower left side, but kept being told there was nothing wrong. Her fear was not of any specific dental procedure or needles or what one would normally think of as fear, rather she was afraid that she was crazy and her mind was playing tricks on her. She was also afraid to get a root canal on a tooth she believed did not need it.

Cases like these have taught me to listen to the patient. Do not assume we know more than they do when it is about what a patient actually feels in their own mouth. I believe that our job, as dentists, is to ask enough questions and allow the patient to find a way to describe their problem. With this personal insight, we can correctly diagnose it and then with our skills, treat it.

TWO INTERESTING STORIES

I have discovered that that no matter where I go, everyone seems to have a dental story to share. Here are two such stories.

STORY #1

I was talking to RG, a business manager, at my car dealership. When he heard that I was a dentist, he told me how fearful he was as a result of an experience he had 24 years previously. He shared with me the following: "I had two teeth pulled by a drunken dentist who forgot to give me Novocaine. My dad heard me screaming and ran into the room. Since my dad was a sergeant, he took the dentist to task and had the dentist put in the brig. It did get all cleared up eventually, but I have been afraid to go to the dentist ever since. The only reason I can go today is because my wife works in a dental office and watches out for me."

STORY #2

A patient and friend of mine shared this dental story. DK remembers being in church with her family when she was a young child and her dad sneezed loudly and when she looked up at him she saw his teeth flying right down the church aisle. She said she immediately felt in her own mouth for her teeth and were reassured that they were still there. She was laughing but was also horrified. She cannot remember how her dad handled it, but she does remember hearing murmurs and people talking all around her pew.

She told me that this memory comes to her occasionally, especially now that she has been undergoing some of her own similar dental treatment.

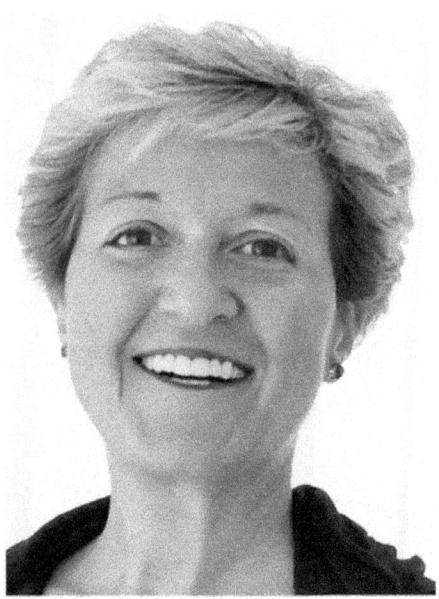

Dear Readers,

I am sure that every one of you has at least one interesting if not horrifying dental story of your own to tell. If you are willing to share them with me, please do so by e-mailing them to me at fatnomorebook@gmail.com.

HAVE NO FEAR OF THE DENTAL CHAIR!

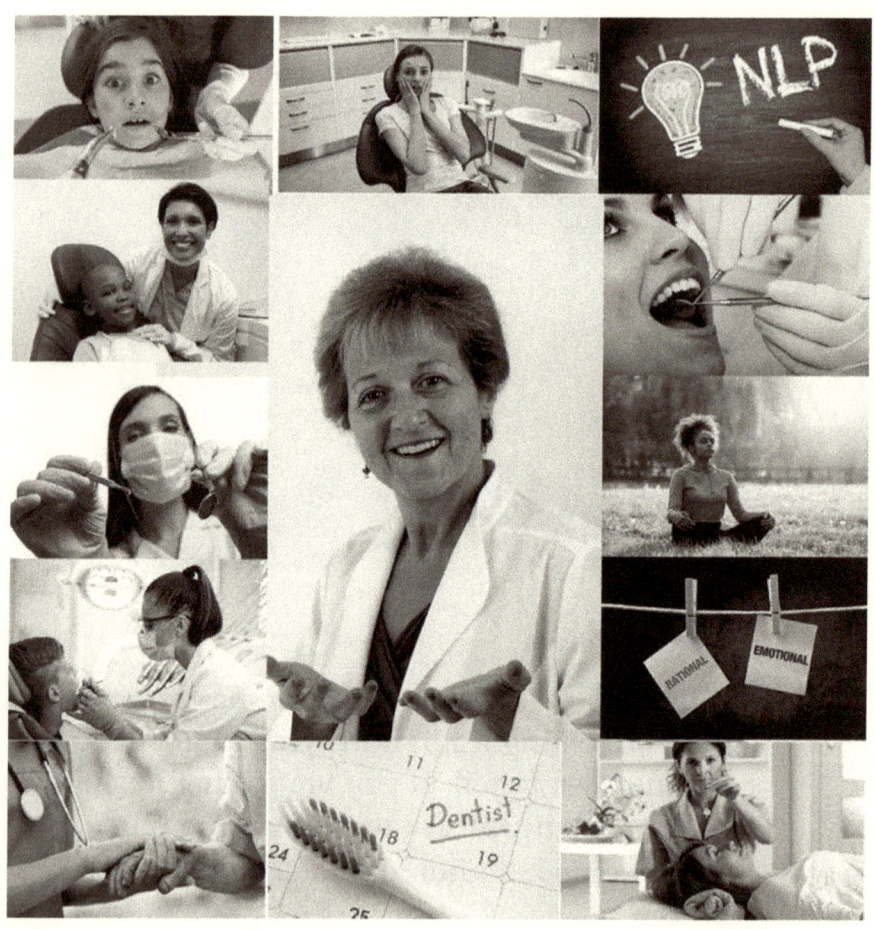

Patient Letters and Testimonials

HAVE NO FEAR OF THE DENTAL CHAIR!

Besides knowing that I have been able to positively change many people's lives by helping them save their teeth and gain confidence that they can make dental care a regular part of their lives, I have had the personal satisfaction of receiving letters from happy patients.

Here are a few of my most memorable ones:

GR writes:

I am so excited about this that I felt it necessary to let other frightened people know there is finally a place even for us. If you are afraid, fear no more.

I am a 71 year old woman who has had a phobic fear of the Dentist all of my life. I have up to now neglected my teeth because of it. I am now forced to do something because chewing has become an issue and I was afraid that I would soon not be able to eat, soooo I bit the bullet and went online to find a fraidy cat Dentist. She is Susan Cushing of Pocasset. From the moment I spoke to her my life has changed. This has just been the most wonderful experience. This woman has put together the gentlest, cheerful and caring staff I have ever encountered. Their whole mission in life seems to be making you comfortable and allaying your fears. There can be an office full of clients and you still feel as if they are there just for you. Everyone has plenty of time to spend with you and this includes the Dr herself. You are never rushed and you just want to be there. The office is cozy and comfortable with no frightening gestures or sounds and nothing is done without explanation or before they are sure you are completely comfortable. There is nothing to fear here. I have now had my 6th visit and I have not dreaded going back at any time. I finally have MY DENTIST. Please don't hesitate to visit this wonderful place.

Gigi

JF writes:

Dear Dr. Cushing and Staff,

This is a long overdue letter in appreciation of your expertise and caring concern for my dental health.

Years ago I entered your office with much trembling and trepidation- I hadn't been to see a dentist "in years" and feared for the worst. Amidst anxiety and tears, I exposed my fears to you, ashamed and really terrified of the position I was in.

Dr. Cushing, you sat me down and empathized with me, reassuring me of the care you would give me- instructing me along the way in what needed to be done and once treatment began, you constantly checked with me on my comfort levels. You even commended me on my "courage" as I went along- from Soft Tissue management to several pullings and crown work.

My mouth is "stabilized" now, and I no longer fear visiting the office. Your staff is very welcoming and caring, too-how much I have always appreciated the "human touch" of a hand holding or the friendly hug.

These years, of paramount importance to me, are the continued support I receive and the awareness I have that I do have a dentist I can trust, who is THERE for me. I do not have to fear the "unknown", the doctor unfamiliar to me, who may or may not be sympathetic to my innate fears. and a doctor who knows what she is doing.

These days, especially, we know the "cost of everything", but do we REALLY appreciate the VALUE of such professionalism?

"Thank you for being you"- my late mother's lovely compliment.

I want this letter to be a "thank you" card and a testament to others of your great ability as a person and a doctor to help all of us to address our fears regarding dentistry. With your sincerity of concern and your knowledge, you have given me the gift of trust- priceless! Sincerely,

Jackie

AF writes:

After years of neglecting my teeth, due to dental fear and bad experiences, I want to express my sincerest gratitude for your caring and unbelievable dentistry.

You and your staff went out of their way to make my recent dental experience comfortable and successful, so far.

I still have many more visits to having my teeth and gums healthy again, but my fear is subsiding and I have you to thank.

With deep appreciation. Sincerely,

Anna Fay

CH writes:

I never thought in 1000 years that I would be writing a letter to my dentist. It took many trips to a sedation website before I saw you as a featured dentist. I played that video over and over, before I finally found enough courage to call your office. Jill patiently listened while I told her about my less than pleasant dental experiences. She then told me I had made the right call and would be comfortable here.

At our first meeting, I could tell that you empathized with me. After many tears, sweaty palms and deep breaths I made it through.

I also could not have felt more at ease with Laura. She explained everything and said we did not have to do everything in one visit. To my amazement we did.

My family has been worried about my health because I neglected my teeth for so many years. I can't thank you and your staff enough for all the comforting words and actions. I no longer turn away when people speak about going to the dentist. I just tell them I have the best dentist!!!

Kindest Regards.

Carole

MS writes:

Dear Dr. Cushing and Staff,

I am sorry that it took me so long to send you all my sincerest thanks for taking such good care of me during my recent dental experiences. I know my dental procedure would probably not have fazed many people but to me it was monumental. From the moment I walked in the door and Jill greeted me I knew I had found my comfort zone!! I know too many people that sounds absurd but to someone who has "fear of the dentist" they can understand. Everyone completely understood my feelings and did not make light of it. Just to know that I can have that "twilight sleep" and go through dental procedures with such ease means the world to me. It had been many years since I had seen a dentist and just to make an appointment was huge. But now knowing I have such a "safe haven" for me is wonderful. Yes, I'll probably still be scared, but I truly know Dr. Cushing's staff is always ready to ease me over the edge. Enough of this epistle, but I just wanted to let you all know how much I appreciate the kindness and compassion shown this "dental chicken." Sincerely,

Martha

P.S. Please feel free to share my thoughts with another "Dental Chicken."

About The Author

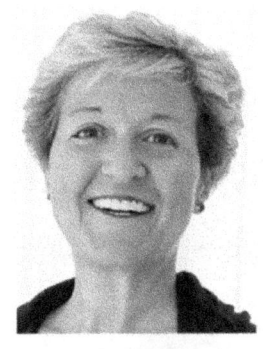

Dr. Susan R. Cushing graduated Cum Laude from Boston College and went on to earn her DMD degree from Tufts University Dental School in Boston, Massachusetts.

She established her first dental practice in Boise, Idaho where she met and ultimately married her husband, Curt. After fourteen years in Boise, she moved back to Massachusetts to be closer to her parents and opened her second dental practice in Pocasset, Massachusetts.

Dr. Cushing published her first book, *Fat No More! The Book of Hope for Losing Weight,* to share her lifelong struggle with obesity and dieting, including all her trials and tribulations and eventual success of losing over 85 pounds and keeping it off for many years. It is a very honest and inspiring message for those fighting the diet/weight battle.

In *Have No Fear of the Dental Chair!,* Dr. Cushing tells the story of her childhood fear of dentists and finding a compassionate dentist who understood her terror and helped turn it around allowing her to find her personal mission of helping patients like herself and becoming an *anti-anxiety advocate*.

Dr. Cushing has been practicing for thirty-four years, using her training and skill helping patients be comfortable while they get their dental care needs accomplished.

In her new book, she offers compassion and understanding for the multitudes of people struggling with dental anxiety and provides a guide to how you can change it.

HAVE NO FEAR OF THE DENTAL CHAIR!

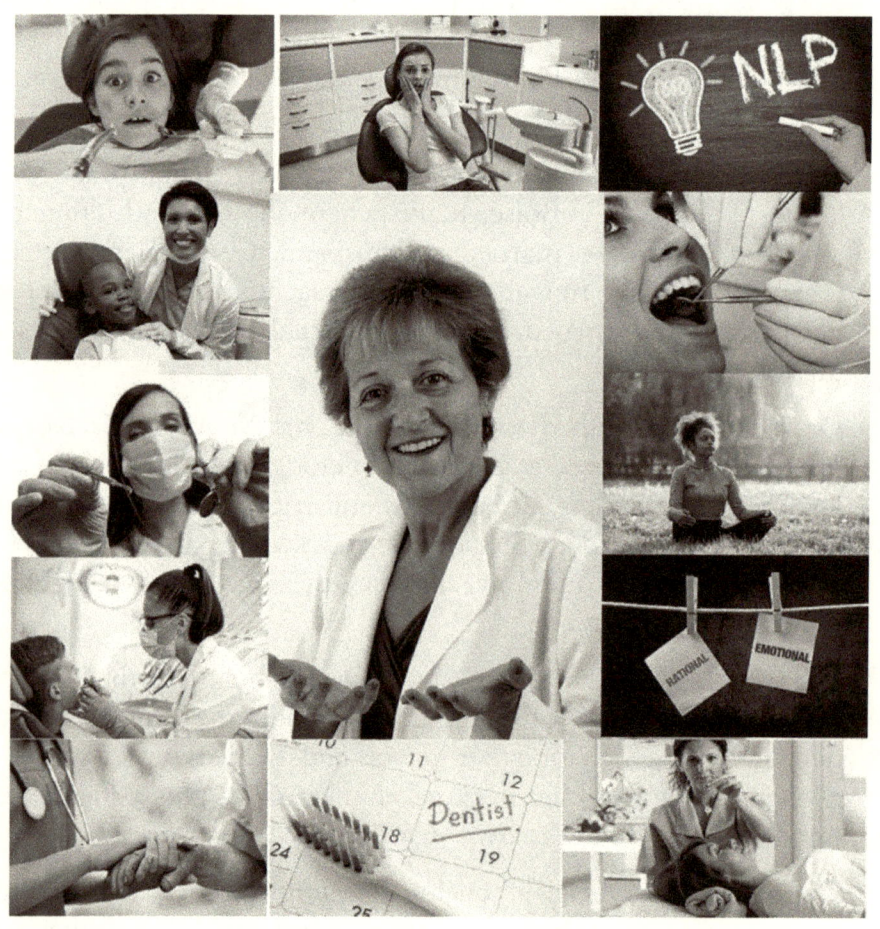

www.ingramcontent.com/pod-product-compliance
Lightning Source LLC
Chambersburg PA
CBHW032108090426
42743CB00007B/277